FRAILTY AND HEART HEALTH

Understanding the Relationship for a Healthier Future

Dr Saifuddin Ekram

Independently Published

ISBN-13: 979-8304768627
Independently Published

Cover design by: Art Painter

Printed in the United States of America

Dedicated to my wife, Monira, whose love, and patience make everything possible

CONTENTS

INTRODUCTION

Frailty and heart disease might sound like two very different problems. One makes you feel weaker and slower over time, and the other affects your heart and blood flow. But the reality is, frailty and heart disease are closely linked—and when they occur together, they can make it much harder to stay healthy and independent as you age.

This book is here to help you understand that connection—and more importantly, what you can do about it.

As people live longer lives, it's not just about counting the years. It's about making sure those years are full of energy, independence, and good health. That's where understanding frailty and heart health becomes so important. Frailty can make your body more tired and less able to bounce back from illness or stress. Heart disease can quietly put pressure on your body, leading to fatigue, shortness of breath, and serious health risks. And together, they can make everyday life harder.

But there's good news: both frailty and heart disease can be spotted early, managed well, and even improved with the right choices and care. That's why this book is written for everyday people—no medical degree needed. We'll cover:

- What frailty really is (and why it's not just "getting old")

- How your heart works—and what happens when it doesn't

- Why these two conditions often show up together

- Simple things you can do at home to stay stronger and healthier

- Tips for eating better, staying active, managing stress, and sleeping well

- How to talk to your doctor and take control of your health plan

This isn't about fear—it's about knowledge and action. Whether you're caring for yourself or a loved one, this book is filled with practical advice to help you live longer, feel stronger, and stay independent for as long as possible.

Because every day matters—and your health is worth protecting.

Let's get started on a healthier future—together.

CHAPTER 1: FRAILTY AND HEART HEALTH

Frailty and heart disease—two words that might seem worlds apart. One conjures images of stethoscopes and cardiac rhythms, while the other reminds us of wobbly knees and the eternal search for that missing pair of glasses. But the truth? These two are more closely intertwined than you would think. Let us dive into why frailty and heart disease are an unbeatable (and not-so-great) duo, and why understanding this connection can pave the way for a healthier future.

1.1 What Is Frailty?

Picture this: Your once sprightly neighbour who used to outpace everyone at the morning walk now struggles to lift their grocery bag. That is frailty. It is not just about feeling old or tired —it is a medical condition that leaves you more vulnerable to life's curveballs, like infections, falls, and even heart disease. It is like when your smartphone battery starts dying after two hours, even though it is supposed to last all day. You are still functional, but everything takes more effort, and you cannot rely on yourself the way you used to.

Frailty is like your body's energy bank running low. Normally, your reserves of strength, speed, and resilience keep you going, but with frailty, those reserves shrink (1). You are more likely to feel weak, move slower, and recover from illnesses at a snail's pace—or maybe slower, like that one snail who refuses to leave your garden. It is not just about getting older. Sure, age is a big player, but lifestyle, chronic illnesses, and even that extra slice of cake (or two) over the years can contribute to the frailty fund. It sneaks up on you, little by little, until one day climbing stairs feels like scaling Mount Everest.

Think of frailty as a spectrum. On one end, you are active, energetic, and tackling your to-do list like a pro. On the other, you are struggling with everyday tasks, and even minor challenges can feel overwhelming. Most of us fall somewhere in between, but here is the kicker: the closer you are to the frail end of the spectrum, the more vulnerable you are to life's curveballs. Even a common cold can feel like being hit by a freight train.

But here is the good news: frailty is not a life sentence. It is not some unchangeable destiny, like your height or your inability to remember where you put your keys. Recognizing it early is like spotting a pothole before you trip over it—it gives you a chance to do something about it. With the right tools, like exercise, good nutrition, and regular check-ups, you can stop frailty in its tracks or even reverse some of its effects. It is like charging that dying phone battery and finally getting through the day without panicking about your charger.

Frailty also loves to team up with other health issues, turning them into bigger problems. If you are already dealing with diabetes mellitus (DM), arthritis, or high blood pressure, frailty might sneak in as an uninvited guest. It makes everything harder—recovering from surgery, fighting off an infection, or just keeping your balance when the dog suddenly decides to sprint past you. But again, this is not about doom and gloom. It is about understanding what frailty is so you can give it a run for its money.

And if you are wondering, "Why does this even matter?" let us get real. Frailty does not just affect the person dealing with it. It impacts families, caregivers, and even healthcare systems. A frail grandparent might need more help at home, extra trips to the doctor, or a longer recovery time in the hospital. It is like a ripple effect, starting small but spreading out to touch everything around it.

So, whether you are the sprightly neighbour or the one who is slowed down a bit, understanding frailty is key. It is not just about adding years to life but adding life to those years. Because let us face it: life's more fun when you can carry your own groceries, chase after the dog, or outpace everyone at the morning walk—even if it is just to get to the coffee first.

1.2 Understanding Heart Disease

Heart disease is like that party crasher who shows up uninvited and wrecks everything. At its core, it is about your heart—the tireless pump that keeps you alive—struggling to do its job. The usual suspects? Blocked arteries, high blood pressure, or that lifelong love affair with junk food.

But let us break it down. Think of your heart as a diligent gardener watering a vast field (your body). Heart disease is like kinks in the hose. Whether it is a full-blown heart attack or an ongoing issue like heart failure, the damage can ripple through every part of you. And just like frailty, heart disease does not play fair. Genetics, lifestyle, and time all conspire to give your heart a run for its money.

Now, let us get into the practical details. Imagine your heart beating roughly 100,000 times a day—yes, even on those lazy Sundays when the most exercise you get is reaching for the remote. That is over 35 million beats a year! It is a non-stop machine, tirelessly working to pump oxygen-rich blood to every nook and cranny of your body. Your brain? Needs the blood. Your toes? Yep, them too. It is a full-body delivery service that never clocks out.

But when heart disease sneaks in, things go haywire. Blocked arteries, for example, act like traffic jams on a major highway. Blood flow slows down, sometimes grinding to a complete halt. If the blockage is severe enough, you might experience the dreaded heart attack (2). Think of it as your heart throwing its hands up and saying, "I quit!"

High blood pressure (3), another culprit, is like a fire hose hooked up to a garden faucet. The pressure strains your heart, making it work overtime. Over the years, this relentless stress can enlarge the heart (not in a good way!) and weaken it. And do not forget about cholesterol (4) —the sticky stuff that loves to build up in your arteries like gunk in an old drainpipe. When too much of it accumulates, your arteries narrow, and your heart struggles to push blood through.

Then there's heart failure (5)—a bit of a misnomer because the heart does not actually stop working. It just becomes inefficient, like a tired old engine that cannot keep up with the demands of the road. Fluid starts to build up, leading to swelling in your legs, breathlessness, and fatigue. It is your body's way of waving a red flag.

Now, here is the thing: heart disease does not discriminate. It is an equal-opportunity troublemaker. Sure, genetics play a role (6). If your family tree is dotted with heart problems, you might have inherited some risk. But lifestyle choices are the real game-changer. That couch-potato lifestyle, smoking habit, or penchant for greasy food? They are like handing heart disease an engraved invitation.

And age? Well, age does not help. The older we get, the more wear and tear our heart endures. It is like a car that is clocked too many miles—the parts start to falter. That is why heart disease and frailty often tag-team in older adults, creating a double whammy of health challenges.

But here is some good news: heart disease is not inevitable. With the right care, you can lower your risks and keep your heart ticking along happily. Exercise, even something as simple as walking, can strengthen your heart and keep those arteries clear. A healthy diet full of fruits, veggies, and whole grains? It is like premium fuel for your body. And regular check-ups with your doctor can catch problems before they spiral out of control.

Heart disease might be a party crasher, but it is one you can keep at bay with some smart choices and a little effort. Your heart is the ultimate team player, and it deserves all the support you can give it. After all, it has been working for you since day one. The least we can do is give it a fighting chance to keep going strong.

1.3 The Hidden Connection Between Frailty And Heart Health

Now here is the kicker: frailty and heart disease are best friends... in the worst way possible. One makes the other worse, creating a vicious cycle (7). A frail body means your heart has to work harder to keep things ticking. On the other side, a weak heart can turn your body frail faster than a melting ice cream cone on a sweltering day.

Let us break this down in simple terms. Your body is like a well-oiled machine—until it is not. When you are frail, it is as if your engine has lost half its horsepower. You are tired, slow, and less able to handle stress. Now, imagine adding a faulty fuel pump (that is your heart disease) to the mix. The machine's performance takes a nosedive, and every hill becomes a mountain.

The science behind this connection is fascinating, though not always fun to live through. Frailty increases inflammation in your body (8)—like a low-grade fever that never quite goes away. Inflammation is no friend to your heart. It stiffens arteries, encourages plaque buildup, and raises blood pressure. Meanwhile, a weak heart struggles to deliver oxygen and nutrients to your muscles and organs, accelerating frailty. It is a vicious cycle where each condition feeds the other, creating a downward spiral of health.

But it is not just biology playing tricks on us. Life with both frailty and heart disease can feel like a series of uphill battles. Picture a frail person with heart disease trying to climb a flight of stairs. For them, it is akin to scaling Mount Everest without oxygen tanks. Even simple tasks like grocery shopping or getting out of bed can feel monumental. And when infections or injuries strike? The body's defences are often too weak to fight back effectively. This is why hospital visits, complications, and yes, even mortality rates, skyrocket when frailty and heart disease join forces.

Here is another layer to the story: mental health. Living with frailty and heart disease can be emotionally exhausting. The constant fatigue, physical limitations, and fear of sudden health crises can lead to anxiety or depression. And guess what? Mental health struggles can further exacerbate physical frailty and heart issues. It is a tangled web where everything—mind and body—is interconnected (9).

But do not lose hope! Understanding this toxic tango between frailty and heart disease is the first step toward breaking the cycle. Prevention and intervention are powerful tools. Exercise, for instance, is like a magic pill—except it is not a pill at all. Regular physical activity strengthens your heart, builds muscle, and boosts energy levels, effectively fighting frailty and heart disease simultaneously. And the best part? You do not need to run marathons. Even gentle activities like walking, yoga, or tai chi can work wonders.

A balanced diet is another superhero in this story. Think of it as premium fuel for your engine. Fresh fruits, vegetables, lean proteins, and whole grains nourish your body and help keep your heart in top shape. Cutting back on processed foods, sugary drinks, and excessive salt can do wonders for both frailty and heart health (10). Remember, what you put on your plate can directly impact how you feel and function (11).

Early interventions are also vital. Regular check-ups with your doctor can catch both frailty and heart disease in their preliminary stages when they are most manageable. Medications, physical therapy, and even social support can play vital roles in improving quality of life. And let us not forget the power of community. Joining a support group or engaging with friends and family can lift your spirits and keep you motivated to stay active and healthy.

Here is the bottom line: Frailty and heart disease may be a terrible duo, but they are not invincible. With the right knowledge and tools, you can fight back. Think of this as a battle where you are armed with exercise, nutrition, and early interventions. By breaking the cycle, you are not just improving your health—you are reclaiming your independence, energy, and zest for life.

So, the next time you hear someone talk about frailty and heart disease, do not just think of them as separate issues. They are two sides of the same coin, and understanding their connection is the key to a healthier, happier future. Stick with us as we unravel more about this complex relationship and explore ways to live stronger and longer.

CHAPTER 2: BIOLOGY OF FRAILTY AND HEART DISEASE

Understanding the composite dance between frailty and heart disease starts with unraveling the biology behind these two fascinating yet challenging conditions. Let us take a closer look—at what makes them tick.

2.1 Frailty: A Marker Of Vulnerability

Imagine your body as a well-built ship. Strong, sturdy, and designed to weather life's storms. But over time, wear and tear start to creep in. Frailty? It is like rust taking hold. It is a clear signal that the ship might not handle rough waters as well as it used to.

But let us be clear—frailty is not just about feeling a bit slower or more tired after a long day. It is your body's way of waving a big red flag and saying, "Hey, things are not as sturdy as they once were. Go easy on me!" At its core, frailty is all about losing resilience—that bounce-back ability that keeps us steady and strong (1).

Think of it this way: when a younger, more robust body encounters a health problem, it is like a trampoline. You bounce right back! But with frailty, it is more like landing on a soggy mattress. Recovery takes longer, and sometimes, it is incomplete. Get sick? It is a steeper uphill battle. Trip and fall? There is a higher chance of something snapping. Living with frailty can want to walk a tightrope—and someone just took away the safety net.

And here is the thing: frailty is not synonymous with aging. We all know that one sprightly grandparent who is outpacing everyone on morning jogs, while a much younger person might struggle to get out of a chair. The secret sauce? Resilience—or, in some cases, the lack of it.

When it comes to heart disease, frailty is like throwing gasoline on a fire. What might be a manageable issue for a fit, resilient person can quickly escalate into something much bigger for someone who's frail. The heart does not just have to work harder—it is doing so with fewer resources to back it up. That is why understanding frailty is about more than just adding years to your life. It is about making those years rich, vibrant, and full of quality.

Frailty is not the end of the story—far from it! It is a call to action to take better care of your ship, patch up the rust, and steer clear of avoidable storms. After all, a well-tended ship, no matter its age, can still sail smoothly into the sunset.

2.2 How The Heart Ages

Your heart is an overachiever. It started beating before you were born and has not taken a vacation since. But, like any long-time worker, it is not immune to aging. Let us break it down.

First, imagine your heart as a well-worn pump. Over the years, it is worked tirelessly to move blood—and with it, oxygen, and nutrients—to every nook and cranny of your body. But with age, even the best pump needs maintenance.

Thicker Walls

As the heart ages, its walls tend to get thicker. Sounds good, right? Like building muscle at the gym? Not quite. This thickening is not like sculpted biceps; it is more like a clogged drain. The thicker walls mean the heart has to work harder to squeeze blood out, kind of like trying to push toothpaste out of a nearly empty tube. It is exhausting for the heart and not very efficient.

Stiff Valves

Next, let us talk about the heart's valves. These little flaps act like doorways, making sure blood flows in the right direction. But over time, these valves can stiffen or get a bit leaky. Think of them as rusty hinges on an old door. They still open and close, but with some creaks and groans, making the whole operation less smooth. This can lead to issues like blood backing up or not getting where it needs to go fast enough.

Electrical System Short-Circuits

Your heart's electrical system is the maestro of its rhythm, ensuring a steady beat. But aging can mess with the wiring. The signals might slow down or misfire, leading to arrhythmias. Translation? Your heart's rhythm might skip a beat or decide to beat too fast or too slow—a bit like a drummer losing the tempo mid-song.

Aging Arteries

Let us not forget the coronary arteries, the blood vessels that feed your heart. Over time, these vessels can become narrower or stiffer thanks to plaque buildup—a process known as atherosclerosis (12). Imagine trying to drink a thick milkshake through a tiny, rigid straw. It is tough! This makes it harder for your heart to get the oxygen-rich blood it craves, especially when it is working overtime.

Less Elasticity, More Pressure

Another thing to watch out for is the loss of elasticity in the heart and its surrounding blood vessels. Think of a balloon that has been inflated and deflated a thousand times. It is just not as stretchy as it used to be. This stiffness makes it harder for the heart to fill and empty efficiently, leading to higher blood pressure and extra strain on the entire system.

Energy Drain

On top of all this, the heart's energy factories—the mitochondria—start to lose their spark. They do not produce energy as effectively as they used to, leaving the heart feeling a bit like an old car running on fumes. It will still get you where you need to go, but it is not winning any races.

Frailty and the Heart: A Dynamic Duo

When you mix an aging heart with frailty, things can escalate quickly (13). Frailty adds another layer of vulnerability, reducing the body's ability to cope with stress. Imagine your heart's trying to run a marathon, but your legs (frailty) cannot keep up. The result? A greater risk of complications, slower recovery from illnesses, and a higher chance of ending up in the hospital.

What Can You Do?

The good news is that you are not powerless. While aging is inevitable (sorry, no time machines yet), taking care of your heart can help it age more gracefully. Exercise, even light activity like walking, can keep the heart stronger and more elastic. Eating a heart-healthy diet—think fruits, veggies, and whole grains—can slow down plaque buildup in the arteries. Regular check-ups can catch valve issues or rhythm problems early, giving you a head start on treatment. So, while your heart might not be the sprightly organ it once was, it is still capable of great things. With a little care and attention, you can keep it ticking along nicely for years to come.

2.3 Shared Pathways: Inflammation, Oxidative Stress, And Beyond

Now for the science-y stuff. Do not worry; we will keep it simple. Frailty and heart disease might seem like separate problems, but they are actually connected through some shared biological pathways (14). It is like they are using the same not-so-great GPS system, and unfortunately, it is leading them down the wrong roads.

Inflammation: Picture inflammation as your body's fire alarm. It is supposed to go off when there's danger, like an infection or injury. But what happens if the alarm gets stuck and keeps blaring? That is chronic inflammation for you. It is like living next door to a never-ending fire drill. This constant state of alert damages tissues, accelerates aging, and creates the perfect storm for both frailty and heart disease. Think of it as a double whammy—your body's natural defences end up working against you.

Oxidative Stress: Meet the villains of our story: free radicals. These tiny troublemakers are like graffiti artists in your body, tagging and damaging everything they touch. Normally, your body has anti-graffiti patrols (antioxidants) to clean up the mess. But as we age, the patrol gets lazy or overwhelmed. The result? Oxidative stress. This imbalance wreaks havoc on cells, contributing to muscle weakness, frailty, and, you guessed it, heart disease. It is like letting chaos reign in a city with no one to restore order.

Hormonal Changes: Aging is a hormonal rollercoaster, and not the fun kind. Levels of key hormones like testosterone and growth hormone drop, and the effects are far-reaching. Muscles shrink, bones weaken, and the energy supply runs low. For frailty, this means less strength and balance. For the heart, it is like asking a tired engine to power a long road trip—it is not going to end well.

Mitochondrial Dysfunction: Mitochondria is called the powerhouse of the cell. These microscopic energy factories keep your body running. But as you age, they start operating like old, sputtering generators. Less energy means muscles get weaker, recovery slows, and fatigue becomes your constant companion. For both frailty and heart disease, this energy crisis spells trouble. It is like trying to charge a smartphone with a frayed cable—you are not getting the full battery life you need.

Chronic Stress: Let us not forget stress, the silent saboteur. Long-term stress floods your body with cortisol, a hormone that, in small doses, is helpful. But too much of it over time wears down your resilience. Think of cortisol as the boss who never stops micromanaging. Eventually, your systems get tired of being overworked, and the effects show up in both frailty and heart disease.

Immune System Decline: As you age, your immune system—your body's defense force—loses some of its sharpness. It is like replacing a SWAT team with mall security. This decline means more vulnerability to infections, slower healing, and a greater risk of chronic diseases, including those affecting the heart.

In a nutshell, frailty and heart disease (15) are not just neighbors—they are messy roommates sharing the same biological apartment. Chronic inflammation sets the place on fire, oxidative stress throws a wild party, and mitochondrial dysfunction cuts the power. Add in hormonal chaos and an overwhelmed immune system, and you have got quite the dysfunctional household.

The good news? Understanding these shared pathways gives us the tools to tackle both issues. By addressing inflammation, boosting antioxidant defences, supporting hormonal balance, and keeping stress in check, we can pave the way for a healthier, more resilient future. After all, it is not just about adding years to life but adding life to years.

CHAPTER 3: RISK FACTORS FOR FRAILTY AND HEART DISEASE

3.1 Aging: The Common Denominator

Aging is like a relentless tide that slowly but surely reshapes the shoreline of your life, regardless of how much you try to hold it back. You cannot stop it, but you can learn to live with it—preferably on your terms. While growing older is a privilege, it also comes with its fair share of surprises, many of which are less than delightful. Frailty and heart disease are two such uninvited guests that tend to tag along as we age. Think of aging as the common thread tying these conditions together, weaving a tapestry of challenges and changes.

As the years roll by, our bodies start to send not-so-subtle reminders that time is marching on. Muscles shrink—it is not that you are losing your biceps overnight, but gradually, what was once firm and strong might start to resemble pudding. Bones lose density, becoming less like steel beams and more like fragile porcelain. And those once-springy joints? They now creak and groan like an old wooden floor every time you move.

But aging is not just about the visible wear and tear. Deep inside, at the cellular level, your body's hardworking little power plants—the mitochondria—start to lose steam. These tiny dynamos are responsible for producing energy, and when they slow down, so does your ability to stay active, strong, and resilient. This decline in cellular energy is one of the key culprits behind frailty, which dreaded condition where even everyday tasks start wanting to climb Mount Everest.

The cardiovascular system also does not escape aging's grasp (16). Your arteries, which should be as flexible as rubber bands, start stiffening up like old garden hoses left out in the sun. Blood pressure rises, forcing your heart to work harder than ever to keep things flowing. Over time, even the most reliable pump can lose its efficiency, and your heart—that incredible, tireless organ—might start struggling to keep up.

Now, here is the curious part: not everyone experiences aging the same way. Some people seem to glide through the golden years like fine wine, becoming more robust and wise with age. They are the ones climbing mountains at 70 or dancing through their 80s. Meanwhile, others face an uphill battle much earlier, dealing with frailty and health problems that seem to arrive before their time. Genetics play a role here—it is like the lottery of life. Some folks hit the jackpot, while others might get a ticket with a few more challenges.

Lifestyle also plays a starring role in how gracefully we age. It is like choosing the fuel for a car: premium or regular. The choices we make about what we eat, how much we move, and how we manage stress all determine whether we are running smoothly or sputtering along.

Staying active, eating well, steering clear of smoking and excessive drinking, and managing stress are like giving your body routine maintenance—it keeps everything running smoothly and efficiently.

Speaking of staying active, there is a simple truth that cannot be overstated: move it or lose it. Physical activity keeps your muscles strong, your joints lubricated, and your heart pumping efficiently. It is not about becoming a marathon runner in your 70s (though, hey, kudos if you do!). Even small, consistent efforts—like a daily walk, some light jogging, or dancing around the living room—can make a big difference.

And let us not forget the importance of laughter and staying socially connected. They say laughter is the best medicine, and science agrees (17). It reduces stress, boosts your mood, and even helps your immune system. Spending time with friends, family, or even your friendly neighborhood dog can work wonders for both your mental and physical health. After all, aging does not have to be a lonely road—it is much more fun with company.

The cardiovascular system—aging's other favorite target—also benefits from a bit of TLC. Your heart might not be as spry as it was in your 20s, but it is still capable of amazing things if you treat it right. Keeping your blood pressure in check, eating heart-healthy foods, avoiding smoking, and staying active are like giving your heart a much-needed vacation from all the heavy lifting.

Interestingly, aging also teaches us the art of adaptation. Cannot lift as heavy as you used to? Try resistance bands instead of dumbbells. Struggling with long walks? Break them into shorter strolls. Aging is less about fighting time and more about working with it. It is about finding new ways to enjoy life while respecting the changes your body is going through.

So, what is the big takeaway here? Aging is inevitable—there is no getting around that. But how do we age? That is where we have some control. By making healthy choices, staying active, and keeping a sense of humour about the whole process, we can loosen aging's grip on our health. After all, if you cannot stop the party crasher, you might as well show them a good time. Here is to be aging gracefully, with a little sass and a lot of heart.

3.2 Lifestyle Factors, Frailty And Heart Disease

Diet, Exercise, and Stress

Regular physical activity, sound nutrition, weight management, and not smoking cigarettes have all been demonstrated to significantly reduce the risk of CVD (18). "You are what you eat" is not just a catchy saying—it is pure science. What you put in your body matters, and if your diet consists of greasy burgers, sugary sodas, and late-night pizza binges, you are basically giving your body the nutritional equivalent of a flat tire. It might get you through the short term, but eventually, things will fall apart. On the other hand, fuelling yourself with wholesome, nutritious foods is like filling up with premium gas. Your body's engine runs smoother, lasts longer, and performs better.

Let us dig into the role of diet. When you overindulge in processed foods and unhealthy fats, your body goes into inflammation overdrive. It is not just about packing on a few extra pounds; it is about creating the perfect storm for diseases like diabetes, heart problems, and —you guessed it—frailty. Low grade inflammation becomes a silent saboteur, weakening your muscles and joints while putting your heart at risk (19).

But here is the good news: you do not have to live on kale smoothies and quinoa alone. A balanced diet filled with colorful fruits, crunchy vegetables, lean proteins, and whole grains can work wonders. Imagine your plate as an artist's palette—the more vibrant and varied the colors, the better. Want a pro tip? The healthier your food looks, the healthier it probably is. (And no, neon-colored gummy bears do not count.)

Next up: exercise. Ah, the fountain of youth! It is free, available to everyone, and requires zero fancy gadgets. Yet so many of us skip it, citing excuses ranging from "I'm too busy" to "I'll start Monday." Spoiler alert: Monday never comes. Exercise is not just about looking good in your jeans; it is about keeping your body functional, strong, and resilient. Think of your muscles as a use-it-or-lose-it deal. The more you move, the less likely you are to lose muscle mass—one of the main culprits behind frailty (10).

Here is the thing: you do not need to become a marathon runner or a gym junkie. Even small efforts count. A brisk walk around the block, a quick yoga session, or playing tag with your kids can make a huge difference. Movement gets your blood pumping, keeps your heart happy, and even gives you an endorphin boost (a.k.a. nature's mood lifter). Endorphins are chemicals produced by the nervous system to cope with pain or stress. They work by binding to opioid receptors in the brain, reducing pain perception and promoting a feeling of well-being. Engaging in physical activity, especially aerobic exercises like running, swimming, or cycling, triggers the release of endorphins, often referred to as a "runner's high". This can lead to feelings of euphoria and reduced anxiety (20). Plus, it is way more fun than staring at a screen all day. Remember, exercise is not punishment—it is self-care in motion.

And now, let us talk about stress. We all know stress—it is the uninvited guest that crashes your peace of mind and overstays its welcome. But stress is not just annoying; it is harmful. Chronic stress has been extensively studied, and there is strong evidence that it leads to elevated levels of cortisol, often referred to as the "stress hormone" (21). Chronic stress floods your body with cortisol, a hormone that is great in short bursts but turns toxic when it sticks around too long. Think of it like a fire alarm that never stops blaring. Over time, this constant state of alarm, i.e., elevated cortisol levels, can disrupt almost all of the body's processes, increasing the risk of health problems such as anxiety, depression, digestive issues, headaches, heart disease, high blood pressure, muscle weakness, sleep problems, weight gain, memory issues. There is an enormous amount of literature on stress and heart disease. These studies show that stressors' contribute to diverse pathophysiological changes including heart attack, chronic heart disease and sudden cardiac death. While stressors set off events, it is less certain that stress directly "causes" them. However, substantial evidence shows that stress negatively impacts the heart, and factors like frailty and lack of resilience influence the extent of these effects (22).

Stress management is not about bubble baths and scented candles (although those can help). It is about finding what works for you. Maybe it is meditation, journaling, or gardening. Maybe it is dancing like nobody's watching or watching comedy shows until you are laughing so hard you cry. The point is to give your brain a break and remind yourself that life is not always an emergency.

Here is where the trifecta—diet, exercise, and stress management—comes together. Picture it as a three-legged stool. If one leg is wobbly, the whole thing topples over. Eating well provides the fuel, exercise keeps the machine running, and managing stress ensures you do not burn out. It is not about being perfect; it is about being consistent.

Smoking

Smoking is like that troublemaking friend who promises fun but secretly wrecks your health behind the scenes. When it comes to frailty and heart disease, smoking is one of the biggest culprits. Let us explore how this habit can wreak havoc on your body and leave your heart and muscles crying out for help.

Frailty: Smoking Saps Your Strength

Smoking has a way of speeding up the aging process. Think of it as a fast-forward button on your body's wear and tear. It reduces blood flow and oxygen delivery to your muscles and bones, leading to weakness and an increased risk of fractures. Your muscles need oxygen to stay strong and active, but smoking deprives them of this essential fuel, leaving you feeling weaker over time (23). Even worse, smoking messes with your immune system, making it harder for your body to repair itself. This can lead to frailty, a condition where small challenges—like a minor illness or fall—can turn into major setbacks.

Heart Disease: Smoking Loves to Break Hearts

Smoking is a big-time villain when it comes to heart health. It damages the lining of your blood vessels, allowing bad cholesterol to stick and form clogs. These clogs make your heart work harder, increasing the risk of heart attacks and strokes (24). And let us not forget high blood pressure. Smoking raises your blood pressure, putting extra strain on your heart. Over time, this strain can lead to heart failure, where the heart struggles to pump blood efficiently.

A Two-for-One Problem

Here is the kicker: smoking does not just cause frailty and heart disease separately—it often links the two. A weak body from frailty struggles even more with heart disease, and a failing heart can make frailty worse (25, 26). It is a vicious cycle, but the good news is you can break it.

The Bright Side: Quit to Thrive

If you are a smoker, quitting is the best gift you can give your heart and muscles. The benefits kick in quickly—your heart rate drops within minutes, and your risk of heart disease starts to decline after just a few months. Over time, your body can repair much of the damage caused by smoking. So, if smoking is that troublemaking friend, it is time to kick them out of your life. Your heart and muscles will thank you, and you will feel stronger and healthier in no time.

Alcohol

When it comes to alcohol, there is often a mix of cheers and concerns. "A little wine is good for the heart," they say, but is it? Let us uncork the facts and pour them out in a simple way.

The Good Stuff

For some people, moderate drinking—think one drink a day for women and up to two for men—might offer heart-friendly benefits. Red wine, in particular, has a buzz around its antioxidants, like resveratrol, which may help protect your heart by reducing bad cholesterol and increasing the good kind. A tiny toast to your arteries? Maybe. Studies suggest that moderate drinking might also help reduce inflammation, which is a win for both your heart and your frailty score (27).

The Not-So-Good Stuff

But here is the hangover to all this good news: alcohol is a tricky friend. Drinking too much—even if you are just "keeping up with the party"—can weaken your heart muscle, leading to a condition called cardiomyopathy. It can also cause high blood pressure, irregular heartbeats, and even strokes (28). And when it comes to frailty, heavy drinking can fast-track muscle loss, worsen balance, and lead to poor nutrition, making you more vulnerable to injuries and illnesses.

Some studies suggest that drinking small to moderate amounts of alcohol might lower the risk of frailty. Interestingly, this link seems stronger in older adults, possibly because they tend to drink less frequently than the general population. However, since this evidence is not very strong, more research is needed to figure out clear guidelines, especially for younger people (29-31). However, alcohol can mess with your diet. When you fill up on beer or cocktails, you might skip nutrient-rich foods that keep you strong and steady. Over time, this can lead to deficiencies in vitamins like B1 (thiamine) and B12, which are important for your nerves and muscles. And let's not forget that alcohol can affect your sleep, making it harder for your body to repair itself—a must for avoiding frailty (29).

How Much Is Too Much?

The magic word is moderation. Excessive drinking can raise your risk for frailty, heart disease, and even dementia. So, if you are reaching for that second glass of wine, ask yourself, "Is this for my health or just because it's there?"

Alcohol, like chocolate or dessert, is best enjoyed in moderation. A glass here and there might keep your spirits high and your heart light, but overindulgence can quickly turn this friend into a foe. If you are living with heart disease or concerned about frailty, it is always a good idea to chat with your doctor about what is best for you.

3.3 Chronic Conditions That Link Frailty And Heart Disease

Some health conditions are like that annoying "friend" who drags you down—the one who always shows up uninvited and overstays their welcome. Chronic conditions are called "chronic" because they do not just go away. You cannot take a week of medicine and expect them to pack up and leave. Instead, they demand consistent care over months, typically exceeding six months (32). Some researchers consider a condition or disease to be chronic if it persists for over a year (33). Chronic conditions such as diabetes mellitus, hypertension, high cholesterol, and obesity do not just stick around; they conspire together, making life much harder. When it comes to frailty and heart disease, these conditions are the troublesome matchmakers—bringing chaos wherever they go (34).

Diabetes mellitus

Let us take a closer look at diabetes mellitus. When it comes to frailty and heart disease, diabetes mellitus often sneaks into the picture as a silent troublemaker. This chronic condition, which affects how the body manages sugar, doesn't just stop at making you rethink your dessert choices; it has a ripple effect on your overall health, including frailty and heart disease (35-37).

How Diabetes mellitus Links to Frailty

Diabetes mellitus can speed up the aging process of your body, making it more likely for frailty to develop. Frailty is not just about feeling tired or weak—it is a combination of physical, mental, and emotional challenges that leave you more vulnerable to health problems. Long-term high blood sugar levels can damage your blood vessels and nerves, leading to issues like muscle weakness, weight loss, and even cognitive decline. These are classic signs of frailty!

For instance, the muscles depend on healthy blood flow to stay strong and responsive. But with diabetes, blood vessels can become damaged, reducing the supply of oxygen and nutrients to the muscles. Over time, this can make it harder to lift heavy groceries or even get up from a chair. And do not get us started on the energy drain—it is like running on a half-charged battery most of the time.

The Heart-Diabetes-Frailty Trio

Now, let us add heart disease into the mix. Diabetes is a major risk factor for heart disease because it causes inflammation and damages the walls of blood vessels, making it easier for fatty deposits to clog them. This not only increases your chances of a heart attack or stroke but also puts extra stress on your heart, especially if frailty has already weakened your body.

When frailty and diabetes team up, your heart faces a double whammy. Weak muscles and reduced energy levels from frailty mean your heart has to work harder to keep your body running. Add diabetes-related complications, and it is like asking your heart to sprint a marathon every day—no wonder it is overworked!

Breaking the Cycle

The good news? You can fight back. Managing blood sugar levels through a healthy diet, regular exercise, and medications prescribed by your doctor is key. Plus, staying active and eating well can help combat frailty and keep your heart in shape. Think of it as teamwork between you and your body—when one part is supported, the whole system thrives. So, diabetes mellitus does not have to take control of your life, but understanding its connection to frailty and heart disease can empower you to make better choices. By managing diabetes and staying proactive about your health, you can break this vicious cycle and live with strength, energy, and a healthier heart.

Hypertension

Next up: hypertension, also known as high blood pressure. Picture your heart as a balloon that is constantly being overinflated. Sure, it might hold up for a while, but eventually, something has got to give. Hypertension forces your heart and arteries to work harder than they should. Over time, this relentless pressure causes wear and tear, leading to heart disease. But that is not all. High blood pressure can sap your energy and limit your physical ability, nudging you closer to frailty's doorstep. For both frailty and heart disease, hypertension is a major player, and understanding its role can help us better manage and even prevent these conditions (38).

The Silent Troublemaker

Hypertension is often called the "silent killer" because it does not usually come with obvious symptoms. However, it puts a lot of strain on your heart and blood vessels, much like trying to water your garden with a hose that is being pinched—it increases the pressure and eventually causes wear and tear. Over time, this strain can lead to a cascade of health issues, from thickened heart walls (a condition called left ventricular hypertrophy) to clogged arteries (atherosclerosis). These issues set the stage for heart disease, including heart failure, heart attacks, and strokes (39).

The Hypertension-Frailty Connection

How does hypertension relate to frailty? While there's limited information on how common hypertension is among frail elderly patients and its link to frailty, recent studies suggest a strong connection (40). Hypertension is more prevalent in frail older adults and is notably associated with frailty. Frailty makes the body more vulnerable to stressors, and high blood pressure adds to the burden. Long-term hypertension can damage small blood vessels in the brain and muscles, reducing blood flow and nutrients to these areas. This can lead to muscle weakness, slower movements, and cognitive decline—classic signs of frailty.

Breaking the Cycle

The good news is, managing hypertension can help reduce the risk of both heart disease and frailty. Lifestyle changes such as eating a healthy diet, reducing salt intake, staying active, and managing stress can work wonders (41). Medications may also be prescribed to keep blood pressure in check. So, think of hypertension as a leaky roof—if you fix it early, you can save your house from major damage. Likewise, keeping blood pressure under control can prevent frailty and heart disease from taking over your life. It is all about taking small, consistent steps toward a healthier future.

Obesity

And then there's obesity. Let us get one thing straight—obesity is not just about appearance. It is about carrying an extra load that your body was not designed to handle. It is like wearing a heavy backpack 24/7. This excess weight increases inflammation, puts your heart under strain, and makes even simple movements feel like a workout. Over time, this extra pressure sets the stage for both frailty and heart disease (42, 43). Let us unpack this!

Obesity and the Heart

Your heart is like the engine of your body, pumping tirelessly to keep you going. When you carry extra weight, it is like driving a car uphill nonstop—it works harder than it should. Over time, this strain can lead to high blood pressure, diabetes, and heart diseases like coronary artery disease or heart failure (44). It is no surprise that obesity is a major risk factor for these conditions.

Obesity and Frailty

Now, here is the twist: you would think someone with extra weight would not face frailty, which is often associated with being thin and weak. But obesity can also lead to frailty, especially when the excess fat is paired with muscle loss, a condition called "sarcopenic obesity" (43, 45). This can make walking, standing, or even climbing stairs feel like scaling a mountain.

The connection between obesity, frailty, and heart disease forms a bit of a vicious circle. Heart disease can reduce your ability to exercise, leading to weight gain and muscle loss. Similarly, frailty can make it harder to stay active, worsening heart health and increasing obesity risk. It is like a merry-go-round you cannot get off—except it is not merry at all!

Breaking the Cycle

The good news? Small steps can lead to big changes. Focus on heart-healthy eating (think more veggies, fruits, and whole grains) and aim for regular activity that matches your ability. Even a short daily walk can help reduce the burden on your heart, improve muscle strength, and keep frailty at bay. By addressing obesity early, we can not only protect our hearts but also maintain the vitality needed for a fulfilling life. Think of it as lightening that overpacked suitcase—you will move through life much more smoothly!

Dyslipidemia

Dyslipidemia may sound like a big, complicated word, but it boils down to something many of us are familiar with: having the wrong balance of fats (lipids) in your blood. Think of it as an unbalanced diet for your arteries. Too much of the "bad" cholesterol (low density lipoprotein, or LDL) and too little of the "good" one (high density lipoprotein, or HDL) can spell trouble for your heart and, as research suggests, may also play a role in frailty (46-48).

How Does Dyslipidemia Affect Your Heart?

When LDL cholesterol builds up in your blood vessels, it is like a traffic jam on the highway—blood flow slows down, and your heart has to work harder to pump blood. Over time, this can lead to heart disease, including heart attacks and strokes. HDL cholesterol, on the other hand, acts like a cleanup crew, carrying bad cholesterol away from the arteries. When the balance between these two gets out of whack, the risk of heart problems goes up (46).

You might be wondering, "What does this have to do with frailty?" But dyslipidemia does not just harm your heart; it can affect your muscles, energy levels, and even your immune system, all of which are crucial to staying strong and independent. Studies suggest that high LDL cholesterol and low HDL cholesterol levels are linked to inflammation in the body. Chronic inflammation is like a slow-burning fire—it gradually damages tissues and can accelerate the aging process. This not only contributes to heart disease but also makes it harder for your body to recover from stress, increasing your risk of frailty (8, 19).

What Can You Do About It?

The good news is that you can take steps to tackle dyslipidemia and protect both your heart and your overall strength. Eating a heart-healthy diet rich in fruits, vegetables, whole grains, and healthy fats (like those from fish and nuts) can help. Regular physical activity, even something as simple as a brisk walk, can work wonders to balance your cholesterol levels. And if needed, medications like statins can help get those numbers in check. So, think of your cholesterol levels as a foundation for good health. Keeping them in balance not only lowers your risk of heart disease but also helps you stay stronger and more active as you age. So, next time you are making choices about what to eat or how to spend your afternoon, remember—you are not just protecting your heart; you are building a stronger, healthier future.

Chronic Arthritis

Arthritis, frailty, and heart disease - if you think about them, they are like the unwelcome guests who show up at the same party, and suddenly it is not so fun anymore. But understanding how they interact can help us navigate their impacts and live healthier lives.

Arthritis: The Achy Joints Conundrum

First up, we have arthritis. It is that pesky condition that makes your joints feel like they have rusted over. The most common types are osteoarthritis, which wears down the cartilage, and rheumatoid arthritis, an autoimmune condition where your body decides to attack its own joints. Neither of these is fun at all. Now, arthritis does not just stay in its lane. It can lead to reduced physical activity because, let us be honest, who wants to move when everything hurts? And this is where frailty starts to creep in (49).

Frailty: The Body's Slowdown Button

Frailty is like the body's way of hitting the slow-motion button. It is a condition that makes you more vulnerable to stressors because of reduced strength, endurance, and overall physiological function. When arthritis makes moving painful, you're less likely to stay active, which can accelerate frailty (50). Less activity means weaker muscles and bones, leading to a vicious cycle of decline.

Heart Disease: The Heart's Silent Struggle

And then there's heart disease (51), the sneaky troublemaker. When frailty sets in, it does not just affect your muscles and bones. It can also impact your cardiovascular system. A weaker body means your heart has to work harder to pump blood, and if you have got arthritis making you less active, your heart does not get the exercise it needs either.

The Interconnected Trio

Here is how it all ties together:

Reduced Activity: Arthritis pain leads to reduced physical activity.

Increased Frailty: Less movement means faster progression of frailty.

Heart Strain: Frailty can exacerbate heart disease by putting more strain on the heart.

Additionally, certain types of arthritis, due to their pathophysiology, can have direct effects on the heart, such as rheumatoid arthritis or systemic lupus erythematosus.

Understanding this trio's relationship helps us find ways to break the cycle. Regular exercise, even if it is low-impact like swimming or walking, can keep the body moving. It helps manage arthritis pain, slows down frailty, and gives the heart a gentle workout. Eating a balanced diet, avoiding smoking, and managing stress are also crucial.

By staying proactive and working with healthcare professionals, we can manage arthritis, frailty, and heart disease better, leading to a healthier and more enjoyable life.

Chronic Kidney Disease (CKD)

Chronic kidney disease (CKD), another player in this game, brings its own unique set of challenges. CKD is not just about tired kidneys; it is like a domino effect, sending ripples through your entire body, impacting your heart and frailty. Let us unpack how these three—CKD, frailty, and heart disease—are surprisingly connected. When your kidneys are not working properly, toxins build up in your blood. This can lead to high blood pressure, anemia, and a host of other problems. It is like a domino effect—one issue leads to another, and before you know it, frailty and heart disease are knocking at your door (52, 53).

CKD and Frailty: The Energy Drain

Your kidneys do more than make you pee! They filter waste, balance minerals, and keep your blood pressure in check. When they do not work well, your body struggles. CKD can leave you feeling zapped of energy, weaker, and more vulnerable. Frailty sneaks in like an uninvited guest, bringing its trademark symptoms: muscle loss, fatigue, and unsteady walking. This is not just aging; it is a bigger storm brewing.

People with CKD often lose vital muscle mass and struggle with inflammation—two big culprits in frailty. Imagine trying to run on an empty gas tank; that is your body on CKD-induced frailty.

CKD and Heart Disease: A Risky Partnership

CKD does not just affect frailty; it has a not-so-secret love-hate relationship with your heart. Diseased kidneys can mess with your blood pressure and cause fluid to build up, making your heart work overtime. Over time, this leads to heart disease—think heart failure, arrhythmias, or clogged arteries.

To add fuel to the fire, CKD can disrupt calcium and phosphorus balance, leading to hardened arteries. It is like trying to pump syrup through your veins instead of water. No wonder the heart struggles!

The Triple Threat

When CKD, frailty, and heart disease team up, it is a triple threat. Frailty weakens your resilience to fight illnesses, while heart disease increases your risk of complications. It is like juggling flaming torches—dangerous and exhausting. But the good news? Recognizing this trifecta can help you take control.

Chronic Obstructive Pulmonary Disease (COPD)

Then we have chronic obstructive pulmonary disease (COPD). COPD is a long-term lung condition that makes breathing harder. It is like trying to get enough air through a straw while walking uphill. This constant struggle for breath can set off a domino effect that impacts your heart and overall health. Living with COPD can leave you feeling tired and weak. This happens because your body is not getting enough oxygen, making everyday activities feel like running a marathon. The lack of oxygen strains your heart and leaves you feeling tired and weak (54-57). Muscle weakness, weight loss, and a general lack of energy—classic signs of frailty—often follow. It is like your body's battery is running low, and the charger is not working fast enough. What is more, COPD often brings flare-ups, or exacerbations, which can knock you off your feet— literally. These flare-ups can lead to hospital stays, loss of muscle strength, and slower recovery times, pushing you closer to frailty.

COPD and heart disease are like two neighbors who cannot seem to keep their problems to themselves. COPD puts extra strain on the heart, especially the right side, because it has to work harder to pump blood through damaged lungs. This can lead to conditions like pulmonary hypertension or even heart failure. Additionally, the inflammation from COPD is not just limited to the lungs—it spreads throughout the body, including the blood vessels. This inflammation can accelerate plaque buildup, raising the risk of heart attacks and strokes. Think of it as rust spreading from one part of a car to another—except the car is your body.

When COPD, frailty, and heart disease team up, the challenges multiply. Frailty makes it harder to recover from COPD flare-ups or heart problems. Meanwhile, COPD makes physical activity—a key ingredient in combating frailty and keeping your heart healthy—more difficult. It is a vicious cycle, but not an unbeatable one!

Managing COPD, improving fitness, and eating a heart-healthy diet are powerful tools to break this cycle. Pulmonary rehabilitation, for example, is like physical therapy for your lungs and body—it can improve your strength, energy, and quality of life. In short, while COPD may seem like a big bully, with the right care and support, you can manage its effects and keep frailty and heart disease at bay.

Chronic Conditions, Frailty and Heart Disease: The common thread

The common thread here is inflammation—a not-so-silent troublemaker that links these chronic conditions to frailty and heart disease (8). Inflammation is your body's natural defense mechanism, but when it is constantly activated (thanks, chronic diseases!), it turns into an internal wildfire, damaging tissues and organs.

So, what can you do about it? The good news is that many of these chronic conditions are manageable. It starts with regular check-ups. Think of your doctor as a detective, piecing together clues about your health. Early detection can make a huge difference. If you have diabetes, keep an eye on your blood sugar levels. If hypertension is your nemesis, monitor your blood pressure. And if you are battling obesity, know that even small changes in weight can lead to big health benefits.

Medication can also be a game-changer. These tiny pills might not seem like much, but they are powerful tools in keeping chronic conditions under control. Whether it is insulin for diabetes, beta-blockers for high blood pressure, or statins to lower cholesterol, following your doctor's advice can help you stay ahead of the curve.

And let us not forget lifestyle changes. Eating better does not mean surviving on kale and water. It is about finding a balance that works for you. Swap out that greasy burger for a grilled chicken sandwich. Add some veggies to your plate. And for the love of your heart, drink more water and less soda. Exercise, too, is a must. You do not have to run marathons—a brisk walk, dancing in your living room, or even gardening can do wonders for your health.

Stress management is another piece of the puzzle. Chronic stress is like a leaky faucet, slowly draining your health. Find what helps you unwind—whether it is yoga, meditation, or laughing at your favorite sitcom. Every little bit helps.

By understanding the role chronic conditions play in frailty and heart disease, you are arming yourself with knowledge. And knowledge is power—the kind that helps you make better choices, live healthier, and keep those annoying conditions in check. So, take control today because a healthier future is waiting for you.

CHAPTER 4: CVD, SURGERY AND FRAILTY ASSESSMENT

4.1 Frailty, Heart Attack And Stroke

Imagine your body as a house. A solid foundation keeps it sturdy through the years, no matter how many storms roll through. But what happens when cracks start forming? Rain seeps in, wood rots, and before you know it, the whole structure is at risk. Frailty is like spotting those cracks early—it is your body's way of whispering, "Hey, take care of me!" And when it comes to heart attacks and strokes, frailty is like the ultimate early warning system.

So, how does frailty cause these cardiovascular events? It is not magic; it is biology. Frailty often brings its gang of troublemakers: chronic inflammation, sluggish circulation, and oxidative stress. These are like termites in the walls of your house, slowly but surely weakening the structure. For your heart and blood vessels, this means more wear and tear, and less ability to bounce back from stress.

The link between frailty and cardiovascular risks has been cemented by research. Large studies show that frail individuals are far more likely to experience heart attacks or strokes, even when they do not have obvious red flags like sky-high cholesterol or blood pressure (58). Why? Because frailty reflects the overall "wear and tear" on your body—a behind-the-scenes look at your heart's capacity to handle the unexpected.

One reason frailty is such a powerful predictor is that it does not happen overnight. It is a slow and sneaky process. You might lose a bit of muscle strength here, feel a little more fatigued there, and suddenly your body is working harder to do the basics—like pumping blood efficiently. Think of it as trying to drive a car with a leaky fuel tank. Sure, the car might still run, but it is burning energy faster and not performing at its best.

Doctors are now realizing that frailty assessment is not just a "nice-to-know" thing; it is a game-changer for prevention. Catch frailty early, and you have a chance to fine-tune your health strategy. Maybe you add more protein to your diet to build muscle or start a low-impact exercise routine to improve circulation and endurance. Sometimes, the solution is as simple as prioritizing rest to avoid burnout.

Now, here is the twist: Frailty is not a life sentence. Yes, it is a sign that your body needs extra care, but it is also an opportunity—a guide to better health. The human body is incredibly adaptable, even in later years. With the right steps, you can regain strength and resilience, reducing your risk of cardiovascular events in the process.

So, what is the takeaway here? Frailty might sound scary, but it is really a heads-up from your body—a chance to course-correct before bigger problems arise. And when it comes to heart attacks and strokes, that early warning can make all the difference. Think of frailty as a guide, not a verdict. It is pointing you toward a healthier path, where small changes today can lead to big rewards tomorrow. After all, houses with a little maintenance can stand strong for decades, and so can you!

4.2 Frailty, Surgery And Recovery

Let us dive deeper into frailty's role in surgery, but first, picture this: you are a trusty old car heading into the shop for a major repair. If your tires are bald, your engine sputters at every stoplight, and your headlights flicker like a haunted house, the mechanic's job gets a whole lot harder. Frailty is the human equivalent—it does not make surgery impossible, but it definitely makes it more complicated.

When frail individuals face surgery, their risks multiply (59) like rabbits. It is not just the scalpel work; it is the body's ability to rally for recovery. Think of it like patching a leaking roof during a thunderstorm—possible, but slow, messy, and with a higher chance of things going wrong. Research shows frail patients are more likely to face complications such as infections, delayed wound healing, or even setbacks like pneumonia or heart failure (60). In fact, prolonged hospital stays and readmissions are common (60), turning what should have been a quick pit stop into an extended stay in the repair shop.

Why Frailty and Surgery Do not Always Play Nice

What is the big deal? Well, frail bodies often lack the reserves needed to cope with the stress of surgery. Imagine running a marathon with an empty fuel tank—you would collapse halfway through. Frail patients often have less muscle strength, reduced energy, and slower metabolisms, making even routine recovery tasks—like getting out of bed or taking a deep breath—a Herculean effort.

There is also the anesthesia factor. Surgery often feels like the easy part; it is waking up afterward that can get dicey. Frailty affects how the body processes anesthesia, making it harder to shake off the grogginess or avoid complications like delirium. And let us not forget the immune system, which in frail individuals might be waving a tiny white flag instead of charging into battle against potential infections.

The Silver Lining: Prehabilitation

Here is the good news: prehabilitation is rewriting the playbook for frail patients facing surgery. Think of it as boot camp for your body—a few weeks of preparation that can make all the difference. Studies show that even simple interventions like improving your diet, doing light resistance exercises, and practicing deep-breathing techniques can help frail patients build strength (61-63).

Nutrition plays a starring role here. If frailty is the leaking roof, good nutrition is the duct tape holding things together until a proper fix is in place. Adding protein-rich foods, hydrating like you are training for a marathon, and even taking specific supplements under a doctor's advice can work wonders. Pair that with low-impact exercises—think gentle yoga, swimming, or short walks—and suddenly your body feels less like a rickety old car and more like a classic vehicle that just needed some TLC.

Even mindfulness training is getting its time in the spotlight. Reducing stress before surgery can improve both mental and physical outcomes, so deep breathing, meditation, or even a few sessions with a counsellor can help frail individuals feel more prepared and less like a deer in headlights.

Frailty Assessments: A Peek Into the Future

Doctors now use frailty assessments as a kind of surgical crystal ball. These assessments measure things like grip strength, walking speed, and how easily someone can get up from a chair. It is like checking a car's oil levels, tire pressure, and brake pads before a road trip—it does not guarantee smooth sailing, but it sure helps avoid nasty surprises.

Armed with these assessments, healthcare teams can tailor surgery plans to individual needs. Maybe the operation is scaled back slightly, or extra recovery time is built into the schedule. Sometimes, doctors might recommend delaying surgery for a few weeks to give prehabilitation a chance to work its magic. It is all about going in prepared, like packing a first aid kit before a camping trip.

Teamwork Makes the Dream Work

Frailty might raise red flags, but it is far from a death sentence for surgical success. With the right care plan, even frail individuals can bounce back beautifully. The secret sauce? Teamwork. Surgeons, anaesthesiologists, physical therapists (PTs), occupational therapists (OTs), dietitians, nurses and—most importantly—the patients themselves work together to stack the odds in favor of recovery.

For patients, it is about taking ownership of their health. Prepping for surgery is not just about showing up on the day—it is about putting in the work beforehand. For doctors, it is about listening, planning, and treating each case as unique. And for caregivers and families, it is about being the pit crew that keeps the engine running smoothly.

So, while frailty and surgery might seem like an odd couple, they do not have to be adversaries. With a little planning, a lot of teamwork, and a sprinkle of determination, even frail individuals can cruise through surgery and recovery, leaving their health storms in the rearview mirror.

4.3 Frailty Scales And Risk Assessment

Here is a question for you: How do you measure frailty? It is not like stepping on a scale or slapping a cuff on your arm for blood pressure. Frailty is a bit trickier—like trying to gauge how wobbly a table is before setting your finest China on it. Thankfully, scientists have taken the guesswork out of it with some pretty smart tools. Think of these as blueprints for your body's foundation. Let us dig in.

Fried Frailty Phenotype: The Big Five

One of the most popular ways to measure frailty is the Fried Frailty Phenotype (FFP) (1). It is straightforward and focuses on five big signs that scream, "I might need some TLC!" These are:

Unintentional weight loss: Dropping pounds without trying sounds great in ads, but in reality, it is often a red flag.

Exhaustion: You are not just tired; you are running on fumes.

Weakness: Your grip strength is so low, even opening a pickle jar feels like a Herculean task.

Slowness: Forget about sprinting; just walking at a normal pace feels like trekking through molasses.

Low physical activity: Couch potato mode, but not by choice.

If you check three or more of these boxes, congratulations—you are officially frail. If you exhibit one or two of these features, you are considered pre-frail. Think of pre-frailty as a yellow warning light on your health dashboard. It is not quite the red "danger" light of full-blown frailty, but it is a sign that you need to pay attention. Pre-frailty is a stage where your body is starting to show signs of becoming frail but has not quite gotten there yet. It is like being on the edge of a cliff, but you have not fallen off. Someone who is not frail should have none of these features. But do not let the label get you down. Think of it as getting a treasure map. It does not mean you are stuck; it just points out where you need to start digging to find your health gold.

Frailty Index: Counting Deficits

Next up is the Frailty Index (FI), which is like a health scorecard (64, 65). Instead of focusing on a handful of symptoms and signs, it looks at the bigger picture. It tallies up all the things that could go wrong—chronic illnesses, mobility issues, memory problems, lab abnormalities, you name it. The more deficits you have, the higher your score.

Imagine taking your car to a mechanic before a road trip. They inspect every little thing —worn tires, a chipped windshield, or a clunky transmission. The FI does the same, but for your body. And just like a higher repair bill means a bumpier ride, a higher frailty score means your health might need extra attention.

Other Frailty Scales: More Tools in the Toolbox

While the Frailty Phenotype and Frailty Index are the stars of the show, they are not the only players in town. Here are a few more tools that doctors and researchers used to measure frailty (66):

Clinical Frailty Scale (CFS): A quick, visual guide that scores frailty on a scale of 1 (very fit) to 9 (terminally ill). It is simple and fast—like judging how ripe an avocado is by squeezing it.

Edmonton Frail Scale (EFS): This one dives into nine domains, including cognition, mood, and even social support. It is like a personality quiz for your health but with way more useful results.

Prisma-7 Questionnaire: A seven-question survey that flags frailty in older adults. It is short, sweet, and effective—kind of like a health speed date.

Frailty Trait Scale (FTS): Focuses on specific traits that add up to frailty, giving a view of your health puzzle.

There are many more tools on the list, but we do not need to mention them all here. Each of these tools has its strengths, and sometimes they are used together for a more comprehensive picture.

Why Frailty Assessments Matter

Now, here's where things get serious—and a little exciting. Frailty measures do not just stop at labeling; they predict risk, especially for cardiovascular events. Studies show that frailty can double or even triple your odds of having a heart attack or stroke (58, 67). Yes, you read that right—triple!

Imagine you are at a casino. If you knew the odds of hitting the jackpot were super slim, you had probably bet conservatively, right? The same logic applies to health. Knowing your frailty score helps you make smarter choices—like prioritizing exercise, eating better, or seeing a specialist sooner rather than later.

Frailty as a GPS for Your Health

Frailty assessments are not here to judge you. They are not the Simon Cowell of health metrics, pointing out every flaw with a raised eyebrow. Instead, they are more like a GPS for your health journey. They tell you where you stand and offer a route to a healthier destination.

For example, if your frailty score is high, your doctor might suggest prehabilitation before surgery or ramping up physical therapy afterward. They might also tweak your medications to reduce side effects or schedule more frequent check-ups. It is all about creating a personalized plan that meets your needs.

The Takeaway

So, do not fear the tape measure, grip strength tester, or questionnaire. These tools are your allies, not your enemies. They turn frailty from a vague concept into something tangible, measurable, and—most importantly—manageable. Remember, frailty is not a life sentence. It is a wake-up call, a chance to take control and chart a new course. With the right measures in place, you are not just surviving—you are thriving. And that is the best kind of treasure map anyone could ask for.

CHAPTER 5: CAN HEART DISEASE LEAD TO FRAILTY?

5.1 Chronic Heart Disease And Frailty

Imagine your heart as a superhero, tirelessly pumping blood day and night to keep you alive. Unlike superheroes, though, it does not wear a cape or ask for applause—it just keeps working. But what happens when that superhero starts losing its powers? Enter chronic heart disease, the kryptonite of your circulatory system. It is like driving a car with a leaky fuel line: inefficient, exhausting, and guaranteed to leave you stranded sooner or later. Chronic heart disease is a broad term that refers to any long-term condition affecting the heart's structure and function. This includes a variety of heart conditions that persist over time and often require ongoing management, such as heart failure, arrhythmias, and valve diseases. Here you should remember about 'coronary heart disease' or 'ischaemic heart disease' (CHD or IHD), which is a major type of chronic heart disease. CHD represents the largest segment within chronic heart diseases. It occurs when plaque (a combination of fat, cholesterol, and other substances) builds up in the coronary arteries, which supply blood to the heart (68-70). Why is CHD the largest group among chronic heart diseases? Well, it is incredibly common. Many people worldwide have risk factors like high blood pressure, diabetes mellitus, high cholesterol, smoking, and a sedentary lifestyle, which contribute to the development of CHD. As a result, CHD accounts for a significant portion of chronic heart diseases.

CHD is not just about your heart feeling overworked or underappreciated. This condition —the result of narrowed or blocked blood vessels—affects how blood flows to your entire body. When the heart cannot pump efficiently, vital organs like the brain, kidneys, and muscles do not get the oxygen and nutrients they need. It is like a city facing rolling blackouts: everything starts to malfunction, one piece at a time.

Now here is where things get personal. Heart disease does not just slow down your heart —it can slow down you. Does that zip you used to have? Gone. The stamina to climb a flight of stairs without feeling like you have summited Everest? Forget it. And that is just the beginning. Over time, the wear and tear from heart disease can chip away at your physical resilience, setting the stage for frailty (7, 71) to move in like an uninvited houseguest.

The Ripple Effect: CHD's Sneaky Sidekick

The relationship between CHD and frailty is like dealing with a troublesome neighbour: one issue spills over and creates another. Let us break it down. CHD reduces blood flow, which means your muscles and organs are not getting their usual energy supply. Imagine trying to cook dinner with a flickering stove—it is frustrating, inefficient, and sometimes dangerous.

Worse still, CHD is often accompanied by chronic inflammation, a sneaky troublemaker in your body. Think of inflammation as the equivalent of a leaky roof—it might seem like a minor issue at first, but over time, it weakens your foundation. This persistent inflammation gnaws away at your muscles, making them weaker and more prone to wasting. It also affects your immune system, leaving you more vulnerable to illness.

To top it off, CHD messes with your energy levels in a big way. Remember the days when you could walk the dog, cook dinner, and still have enough energy to chat with friends? Well, CHD is like a thief that robs you of those reserves. Even simple activities—like brushing your teeth or getting dressed—start to feel like major feats.

Your Energy Bank: Why Every Withdrawal Matters

Let us switch gears and think of your body as a bank account. Every activity—walking, gardening, even laughing—makes a small withdrawal from your "energy account." When you are healthy, your account has enough savings to handle these withdrawals with ease. But when CHD enters the picture, it is like you are hit with hidden fees. You are withdrawing more energy than you are putting in, and soon, you are running on empty.

This "overdraft" leaves you feeling tired, weak, and more vulnerable to frailty. You might notice you are moving slower, feeling less steady on your feet, or needing longer to recover from minor illnesses. It is not just about growing older—it is about your energy economy spiraling out of balance.

The Domino Effect: CHD, Frailty, and Independence

Here is the kicker: when frailty sets in, it does not just affect your physical health—it impacts your whole life (72, 73). Tasks you once took for granted, like cooking, cleaning, or going grocery shopping, start to feel insurmountable. You may begin relying on others for help, which can be frustrating and emotionally draining.

The mental toll of CHD and frailty should not be underestimated either. Feeling constantly tired or dependent on others can lead to anxiety, depression, or a loss of self-confidence. It is like being stuck in a vicious cycle: the less active you are, the weaker you become, and the weaker you become, the harder it is to stay active.

Hope on the Horizon: Fighting Back Against CHD and Frailty

But do not lose heart—literally or figuratively! Understanding the link between CHD and frailty is the first step to fighting back. With advances in medicine, better awareness, and proactive management, you can take charge of your health and reduce the risk of frailty, even if you have CHD.

Lifestyle changes, like eating a heart-healthy diet, staying active within your limits, and managing stress, can help slow the progression of CHD and preserve your energy reserves. And if you are already feeling frail, there are still ways to rebuild strength and independence.

Remember, your heart is still a superhero—it just might need a little help getting its cape back. By treating CHD seriously and addressing its ripple effects, you can protect your energy account and maintain your quality of life. After all, the goal is not just to live longer; it is to live better.

5.2 How Heart Failure Accelerates Frailty

Before examining the relationship between heart failure and frailty, let us break down heart failure in a way that is easy to understand.

Picture your heart as a superhero—let us call it 'Captain Pump'. Captain Pump's job is to keep the blood flowing through your body, delivering oxygen and nutrients to every nook and cranny. But sometimes, Captain Pump starts to struggle. Maybe it is because of years of high blood pressure, clogged arteries, chronic heart disease or other health issues. When this happens, Captain Pump cannot thrust blood as effectively as it used to. This is what we call heart failure. It does not mean that Captain Pump has stopped working altogether—it just means it is not as strong as it once was. As a result, your body does not get all the blood (and oxygen) it needs. This can make you feel tired, short of breath, and cause your ankles and feet to swell up, because fluid builds up when the heart is not pumping well. Heart failure is like when your heart says, "I'm not quitting, but I'm cutting back on hours." It is the sluggish co-worker in the office of your body, leaving everyone else to pick up the slack. This chronic condition, where the heart does not pump blood as efficiently as it should, is not just a heart problem—it is a full-body saga. And when it comes to frailty, heart failure does not just show up at the party; it brings fireworks (74, 75).

If chronic heart disease (CHD) is the gateway to frailty, heart failure is the express train, speeding up the process with multiple stops along the way. Each stop is a challenge—fatigue, muscle weakness, shortness of breath, and even a toll on your mental health. Let us explore this bumpy ride in detail.

Fatigue: The Energy Thief

Fatigue is one of the most recognizable hallmarks of heart failure, and it is a sneaky saboteur. Think about how you feel after pulling an all-nighter—now multiply that by 10 and make it your daily reality. Heart failure causes reduced blood flow, which means your muscles and tissues are not getting the oxygen and nutrients they need to function efficiently.

This crushing exhaustion does not just leave you napping in the middle of the day; it stops you from doing the things you love. Gardening? Too tiring. A walk with friends? Too exhausting. Even climbing stairs can feel like scaling Mount Everest. And here is the kicker: when you stop moving, your body starts losing strength. Muscles shrink, joints stiffen, and reflexes slow. It is a perfect storm, and frailty thrives in it.

The Cascade Effect: When One Problem Leads to Another

Heart failure is the gift that keeps on giving—and not in a good way. One of its hallmark issues is fluid buildup, medically known as edema. Your ankles swell, your legs feel heavy, and walking becomes more of a shuffle. It is like trying to move around with sandbags tied to your feet.

As fluid accumulates, it does not just sit in your legs; it also creeps into your lungs. This makes breathing a challenge, leaving you gasping for air during even the simplest activities, like making your bed or climbing a single flight of stairs. Imagine trying to breathe through a straw while carrying those sandbags—it is no wonder so many people with heart failure lose their zest for life.

What is worse is how these physical limitations rob you of independence. Tasks you used to handle without thinking—cooking, cleaning, shopping—become monumental challenges. Over time, this dependence chips away at confidence and dignity, both of which are vital for staying robust and resilient.

The Brain-Body Connection: Frailty Starts Upstairs Too

Heart failure does not just stop at sapping your physical strength; it takes a swing at your mental health, too. Depression and anxiety are common companions of heart failure, and it is not hard to see why. When your body feels like it is betraying you, it is tough to stay upbeat.

But there is more to it than just feeling blue. Heart failure can also affect your cognition. Remembering names, focusing on tasks, or even planning your day can become harder. Researchers suspect that reduced blood flow to the brain and the chronic inflammation associated with heart failure might be to blame. And when your mind starts to struggle, your body is not far behind—frailty feeds on this brain-body disconnect.

Here is a sobering thought: depression and cognitive decline make it harder to stick to healthy habits, like exercising or eating well, creating a vicious cycle. The less you do, the weaker you get, and the weaker you get, the less you can do. It is a spiral that is hard to stop—unless you know how to hit the brakes.

Breaking the Cycle: Hope for a Healthier Future

The good news? Frailty caused by heart failure is not a life sentence. Understanding how these conditions fuel each other is the first step to breaking the cycle.

First things first, have a consultation with your doctor. They will figure out what is going on and set you up with the right treatment.

But remember, it is not just about the meds—there is plenty you can do to support your own health too. Start with small, manageable changes. Gentle exercises, like walking or chair yoga, can help rebuild strength without overtaxing your heart. Think of it as giving your muscles a pep talk: "You've got this, guys!"

Diet matters, too. A heart-healthy diet rich in fruits, vegetables, lean proteins, and whole grains can reduce inflammation and give your body the fuel it needs to fight frailty.

And do not forget your mental health. Support groups, counseling, or even just talking with friends can ease the emotional burden of heart failure. Sometimes, knowing you are not alone making all the difference.

What We Can Learn

Heart failure accelerates frailty by acting on multiple fronts—it zaps your energy, weakens your muscles, overloads your lungs, and clouds your mind. But it is not an unstoppable force. By taking small, intentional steps, you can keep frailty at bay and regain control of your life.

Remember, heart failure is not your story's ending—it is just a plot twist. With the right mindset, support, and tools, you can write the next chapter as one of strength, resilience, and independence. After all, your heart may have cut back on hours, but you have not!

5.3 Cardiac Rehabilitation And Frailty

If heart disease and frailty are the villains in this story, then cardiac rehabilitation is the superhero who does not just save the day—it gives you the tools to save yourself. Imagine it as a personal health boot camp, customized to help your heart and body stage a comeback worthy of an Oscar.

But let us get one thing straight: cardiac rehab is not about running marathons or morphing into a fitness influencer. It is about meeting you where you are and helping you get where you want to be—stronger, steadier, and with a spring in your step. Whether you are bouncing back from a heart attack, recovering from heart surgery, or managing a chronic heart condition, cardiac rehab is your secret weapon against frailty (76, 77).

Rewiring the Link Between Heart Disease and Frailty

So, how does cardiac rehab break the vicious cycle between heart disease and frailty? First, let us talk about your muscles. Heart disease often makes people feel like they have hit a permanent energy slump, turning activities like climbing stairs or walking the dog into Olympic events. Over time, this lack of activity chips away at your muscle strength, coordination, and balance, leaving the door wide open for frailty to stroll in.

Enter cardiac rehab. Through structured, supervised exercise, it helps rebuild those muscles—literally. We are not talking about pumping iron like a bodybuilder but functional movements that restore what has been lost. Walking on a treadmill, pedalling a stationary bike, or even gentle strength training with resistance bands can help improve blood flow, boost endurance, and increase flexibility. It is like oiling a squeaky hinge—the more you move, the better your body works.

What is even more impressive? Exercise does not just strengthen your muscles—it strengthens your heart, too. A more efficient heart means better circulation and more oxygen delivered to your body, which translates to fewer moments of "I need to sit down before I keel over." It is like upgrading your body's power grid.

More Than Exercise: A Holistic Approach to Staying Strong

But cardiac rehab is not all lunges and leg lifts. It is also about what you put on your plate, how you manage stress, and how you handle life's curveballs. This is where education comes in —a cornerstone of any good rehab program and a holistic approach to staying strong (78).

Imagine you are handed a life manual filled with practical tips: how to whip up heart-healthy meals, decode nutrition labels, and sneak more veggies into your diet. You will learn the ins and outs of stress-busting techniques—like meditation or deep breathing—because stress is not just bad for your ticker; it is a fast track to physical and mental burnout.

And then there's sleep. Ah, glorious sleep! Poor sleep quality often tags along with heart disease, leaving you groggy and irritable. Cardiac rehab teams understand this and provide strategies to improve your shut-eye. Better sleep means better recovery, sharper thinking, and, you guessed it, a lower risk of frailty.

Let Us Talk Mental Health

Now, here is a curveball most people do not see coming: cardiac rehab also has a knack for lifting your spirits. Living with heart disease can want to carry an invisible weight—it is isolating, frustrating, and sometimes downright scary. Depression and anxiety are not just companions to heart disease; they are accelerators of frailty.

Cardiac rehab programs tackle this head-on with counseling and support groups.

Whether it is a one-on-one chat with a psychologist or a group session with others who "get it," you will find tools to cope with the emotional rollercoaster. And once your mental health gets a boost, your physical health often follows suit. It is a win-win for your heart and your head.

The Numbers Do not Lie

You might be wondering, "Does this really work?" Spoiler alert: it does. Studies show that people who complete cardiac rehab programs are less likely to experience debilitating frailty (76, 77). They also have lower rates of hospitalization, better physical function, and longer, healthier lives.

Picture this: fewer falls, less reliance on others to get through your day, and more time spent doing what you love—whether it is gardening, traveling, or chasing your grandkids around. Cardiac rehab does not just add years to your life; it adds life to your years.

A New You, One Step at a Time

The beauty of cardiac rehab is its flexibility. It is not a one-size-fits-all program—it is tailored to you. Whether you are 55 or 85, a walker or a slow-and-steady ambler, there is a plan that fits your pace. The goal is not perfection; it is progress.

And guess what? It is never too late to start. Even if you are already feeling the effects of frailty, cardiac rehab can help slow its progression and, in some cases, even reverse it. Every small step counts, and every effort adds up.

Wrapping It All Up

Heart disease and frailty may be a double whammy, but they are no match for a well-rounded cardiac rehab program. By focusing on the whole, you—your strength, nutrition, mental health, and more—it creates a foundation for resilience that lasts a lifetime. So, let us flip the script. Instead of letting heart disease and frailty call the shots, take the reins. Cardiac rehab is not just about fixing what is broken; it is about building a healthier, happier you—one that is ready to face the future with confidence. Because your heart deserves more than care—it deserves a fighting chance.

CHAPTER 6: FRAILTY AS A CAUSE OF HEART DISEASE

6.1 Why Frailty Increases Cardiovascular Risk

Frailty does not just nudge your independence out the window; it has a sneaky side hustle —putting your heart at risk. While most people think of frailty as something that happens after your heart starts misbehaving, the truth is that frailty can actually pave the way for cardiovascular problems. Picture a two-way street, full of potholes, with frailty and heart disease waving at each other as they wreak havoc on your body (7).

Chronic Inflammation

Let us start with inflammation—the not-so-silent troublemaker. When you are frail, your body tends to have a simmering level of chronic inflammation. It is as if your immune system is a car alarm that will not stop blaring, even when there is no danger. At first, it is just annoying, but over time, it starts to cause real damage.

This chronic inflammation targets your blood vessels, making them less elastic and more prone to blockages. It is like turning your once-smooth arteries into lumpy, bumpy roads where blood struggles to flow. The result? A higher chance of developing heart disease, including those annoying heart attacks and strokes we all want to avoid.

Metabolic Chaos: Frailty's Sidekick

Frailty does not just leave you feeling weaker; it messes with your body's internal chemistry, too. Blood sugar levels go haywire, cholesterol starts acting like a rebellious teenager, and blood pressure spikes or plummets unpredictably. Together, these changes create the perfect recipe for cardiovascular disaster.

Imagine your body as a finely tuned orchestra. Frailty throws the rhythm section off-beat, the brass section starts playing random notes, and suddenly the entire performance falls apart. This metabolic mess makes it harder for your heart to function smoothly, increasing your risk of developing conditions like coronary artery disease.

Inactivity: The Silent Saboteur

Now, let us talk about movement—or the lack thereof. Frailty often leads to reduced physical activity because, let us face it, when your muscles feel like Jell-O, the last thing you want to do is take a brisk walk. But here is the catch: inactivity is one of the worst things you can do for your heart.

Without regular exercise, your heart muscle gets lazy, your circulation slows down, and you miss all the benefits of staying active. Exercise is like a spring cleaning for your cardiovascular system, clearing out clogs and keeping everything running smoothly. When frailty stops you from moving, it is like ignoring a clogged drain—it only gets worse over time.

Stress and the Heart: A Vicious Cycle

Frailty does not just affect your body; it takes a toll on your mind, too. Feeling frail can lead to stress, anxiety, and even depression. And when you are stressed, your heart feels it. Stress makes your blood pressure climb, your heart rate soar, and your blood vessels tighten up like they are bracing for a storm.

The result? A perfect storm of cardiovascular risk factors, all triggered by the mental strain of frailty. It is a vicious cycle: frailty makes you stressed, and stress weakens your heart, which makes you feel even frailer. Breaking this cycle is the key to protecting your heart health.

Breaking the Link: What You Can Do

The silver lining here is that frailty does not have to be a one-way ticket to heart disease. In fact, addressing frailty can have a ripple effect, improving not just your overall health but also giving your heart a much-needed break.

Nutrition: Start with what is on your plate. A diet rich in fruits, vegetables, whole grains, and lean proteins can reduce inflammation and stabilize your metabolism. Think of it as feeding your body the fuel it needs to fight back.

Gentle Exercise: You do not have to run marathons to make a difference. Activities like walking, yoga, jogging, or even gardening can help strengthen your muscles, improve circulation, and keep your heart in good shape.

Inflammation Management: Work with your healthcare team to address chronic inflammation. Whether it is through medications, lifestyle changes, or both, keeping inflammation in check is a key step toward protecting your heart.

Mind Matters: Do not ignore your mental health. Stress management techniques like meditation, deep breathing, or talking to a therapist can help break the stress-heart disease cycle.

Looking Ahead

The link between frailty and cardiovascular risk might seem daunting, but understanding it is half the battle. By recognizing how frailty sets the stage for heart disease, we can take proactive steps to fight back. After all, your heart deserves more than to be caught in frailty's crossfire—it deserves care, attention, and a little bit of love.

6.2 Loss Of Muscle Mass And Cardiac Function

Think of your muscles as the scaffolding that keeps your body upright and moving. Now imagine that scaffolding starting to crumble—not all at once, but bit by bit. That is what happens when frailty tightens its grip. The result is not just weak arms or shaky legs; it is a ripple effect that reaches deep into your chest, impacting your heart—the MVP of muscles.

Let us start with your skeletal muscles, the ones that let you climb stairs, open jars, or hold a yoga pose (even if it is a wobbly tree). These muscles and your heart are besties—more like teammates in a relay race. Your biceps, quads, and core muscles do their part to keep you moving, and your heart keeps them fuelled with oxygen-rich blood. When muscle mass starts to disappear—a condition called sarcopenia (79)—it is like losing half your team in the middle of a game. Your heart suddenly has to play all positions, and trust me, it is not thrilled about it. This extra strain can wear your heart down over time. The harder it has to pump to make up for the loss of skeletal muscle, the more likely it is to lose its own efficiency. Imagine running a marathon with one shoe missing—it is possible, but it is going to cause problems down the road. Over time, this constant overwork can lead to reduced cardiac function or even structural changes in the heart, like a remodel you did not ask for.

But wait, there is more! Skeletal muscles are not just for flexing; they also act as mini-pumps that help blood flow back to your heart. When you take a brisk walk or even wiggle your toes, your leg muscles assist in pushing blood upward against gravity. It is a nifty bit of teamwork. But when muscle mass diminishes, these helpful pumps go offline, and your heart has to take over. No wonder frailty often comes with fatigue and shortness of breath—your heart is stuck pulling double shifts.

Now let us talk about the heart itself. Just because it is smaller than your biceps does not mean it gets a free pass from frailty's effects. Your cardiac muscle is also vulnerable to the same bad influences that chip away at your skeletal muscles: lack of exercise, poor nutrition, and chronic inflammation. These factors can weaken the heart muscle, making it less effective at pumping blood. It is like your heart is going to the gym less often and losing its gains.

Here is the kicker: when your heart struggles, your body struggles too. Poor cardiac function leads to reduced oxygen delivery to the tissues, which further accelerates muscle loss. It is a vicious cycle—a feedback loop of frailty that leaves both your heart and your muscles caught in the crossfire.

But do not despair. The beauty of this interconnected system is that improvements in one area can benefit the whole team. Even small changes to your daily routine can help tip the balance in your favor. Take walking, for instance. A regular stroll does not just stretch your legs—it strengthens them. This reduces the load on your heart and helps with circulation, giving your cardiovascular system some much-needed R&R.

Other options? Swimming is fantastic—it is low impact, gentle on the joints, and great for both your heart and muscles. Or try gardening, which is sneakily effective; all that digging, lifting, and watering works more muscles than you might think. Resistance training is another superstar. Lifting light weights or using resistance bands can help rebuild muscle mass, improving both your strength and your heart's efficiency.

Nutrition matters too. Think of protein as the fuel your muscles need to stay in the game. Foods like lean meats, fish, beans, and nuts are muscle-friendly choices. And do not forget the heart-healthy all-stars: leafy greens, berries, and whole grains. They help reduce inflammation, which is like the sneaky saboteur of both muscle and heart health.

Here is the big takeaway: your muscles and your heart are inseparable partners in your overall health. When one struggles, the other steps in—but only up to a point. By nurturing both through activity, good food, and even just a little TLC, you can keep them working together like a well-oiled machine. It is not about becoming a bodybuilder or a marathon runner; it is about giving your body—and your heart—a fighting chance to thrive. After all, your heart works hard for you every second of every day. Does not it deserve a little help from its friends?

6.3 Frailty And Major Cardiovascular Events

Frailty does not just whisper trouble—it shouts it through a megaphone. If you are frail, you are walking a tightrope over the valley of major adverse cardiovascular events (MACE) (14, 58). These include the heart-stopping trifecta: heart attacks, strokes, and sudden cardiac arrest. Serious stuff, right? But why does frailty seem to hand out free passes to these unwelcome guests? Let us dive in.

Frailty and the Body's Stress Response: The Brittle Rubber Band

Picture your body as a trusty rubber band. When you are healthy, it stretches, bounces back, and handles life's little tugs and pulls without breaking a sweat. But when frailty enters the picture, that rubber band gets brittle and fragile, like one that has been baking in the sun too long. Any big tug—a blocked artery, a sudden drop in blood pressure—can snap it.

Here is why this matters: cardiovascular events are massive stressors (22). They demand your body to mount an all-hands-on-deck response—mobilizing energy, repairing damage, and adapting to the crisis. Frail individuals struggle here because their reserves—the physical and functional equivalent of a rainy-day fund—are already running low. Recovery is slow, incomplete, and often accompanied by complications.

Frailty's Entourage of Health Problems: The Perfect Storm

Frailty does not travel alone. It brings a posse of other health issues, like diabetes mellitus, high blood pressure, and chronic kidney disease. Each of these conditions is already a risk factor for cardiovascular disease on its own. Combine them with frailty, and you have a perfect storm brewing.

Imagine trying to put out a house fire while simultaneously patching up a leaky roof and battling termites. That is what it is like for a frail body handling a cardiovascular event. Each additional condition saps more energy, complicates treatment, and increases the risk of long-term damage.

And that is not all. Chronic inflammation—a hallmark of frailty—plays a starring role. Inflammation fuels atherosclerosis (the buildup of fatty plaques in your arteries), making it more likely for those plaques to rupture and trigger a heart attack or stroke. It is like adding gasoline to an already smouldering fire.

Frailty and Surgical Outcomes: High Stakes in the Operating Room

When it comes to heart surgery or procedures like stenting, frailty is the elephant in the operating room. Surgeons know that frail patients face a rockier road to recovery. Wound healing is slower, infections are more common, and the overall risk of complications skyrockets.

It is not just the surgery itself that is daunting—it is the aftermath. For frail individuals, a hospital stay can lead to deconditioning (loss of muscle strength and physical function), setting off a vicious cycle that is hard to reverse. This is why some doctors hesitate to recommend invasive procedures for frail patients. It is a tough call: the heart problem might need fixing, but the risks of surgery could outweigh the benefits.

But here is the twist: frailty is not an automatic no-go for surgery. With proper preoperative care—think nutrition support, tailored exercise plans, and meticulous management of underlying conditions—many frail patients can navigate surgery successfully. The key is preparation, like stretching before a big run, except this is about prepping your entire body for a major event.

Prevention: Your Heart and Frailty's Worst Nightmare

Now, let us get to the good stuff: what you can do to tip the scales in your favor. Frailty might increase the risk of MACE, but it is not a one-way street. You have the power to strengthen your body and reduce those risks.

Start with the basics

Eat like a heart health ninja: Your plate should look like a rainbow of veggies, lean proteins, whole grains, and healthy fats. Think of it as feeding your body high-octane fuel.

Move it or lose it: Physical activity is not just good for your muscles; it is a lifeline for your heart (80). Walking, swimming, or gentle resistance exercises can work wonders. The key is consistency, not heroics.

Tame the chronic beasts: Conditions like high blood pressure, diabetes mellitus, and kidney disease need to be managed like a well-oiled machine. Keep up with medications, monitor symptoms, and check in with your healthcare team regularly.

Rest and de-stress: Sleep and relaxation are like hitting the "reset" button on your body. Chronic stress and poor sleep can worsen frailty and heart health, so prioritize both.

Even if you are already frail, small changes can have big effects. Research shows that targeted interventions—like supervised exercise programs—can improve strength and resilience, reducing the risk of MACE.

The Wake-Up Call

The link between frailty and cardiovascular disease is a loud wake-up call, but it is also a chance to take action. By understanding the connection, you can make informed choices that protect your heart and boost your overall health. Remember, your body is more adaptable than you think, even when frailty tries to play the spoiler. So, while frailty and heart disease might be tangled in a complicated relationship, the story does not have to end in heartbreak. With a focus on prevention, resilience, and proactive care, you can rewrite the script and aim for a healthier, brighter future. Start early, the sooner, the better.

CHAPTER 7: IDENTIFYING FRAILTY

7.1 Physical Markers Of Frailty

Imagine this: You are at a family gathering, and your aunt, who used to out-dance everyone at weddings, now struggles to carry a small plate of food. Or your uncle, known for his hearty appetite, suddenly skips dessert and has pants that hang loose around his waist. What is going on? These could be physical markers of frailty—your body's way of quietly waving a white flag.

Weakness: The Shrinking Muscle Mystery

Muscle weakness might sneak up on you, but it does not have to be a mystery. It is like an old rubber band—once snappy, now stretched out and tired. Frailty weakens the muscles you need to do everyday tasks: lifting groceries, climbing stairs, even opening that stubborn pickle jar. Strength fades because of inactivity, aging, or health conditions that steal your energy.

Imagine your muscles as a well-oiled machine that needs regular maintenance to function at its best. Over time, if that maintenance is neglected, parts start to rust and break down. Similarly, without regular physical activity, your muscles lose their strength and become less efficient.

How can you spot it? Pay attention to grip strength (cannot unscrew that bottle anymore?), struggles with balance, or an overall slowdown in movements. Even tasks that once seemed effortless, like standing up from a chair or walking across the room, can become daunting challenges.

Weight Loss: Not the Good Kind

Weight loss is not always worth celebrating, especially when it is unintentional. Think of it as a bank account. When frailty sets in, your body starts withdrawing reserves—muscle mass and fat—without your permission. Sudden weight loss can also mean your body is not getting enough fuel to run its basic machinery.

Let us paint a picture: Your body is a car, and food is the fuel. If you do not fill up the tank, the car cannot run properly. Similarly, without adequate nutrition, your body starts to break down its own tissues to get the energy it needs. This can lead to a decrease in muscle mass, making you weaker and more prone to fatigue.

Recognizing this means checking your appetite. Is food losing its appeal? Are clothes fitting differently? These subtle signs are worth noting because losing weight in frailty often goes hand-in-hand with losing strength and energy.

Exhaustion: The Unshakable Fatigue

This is not your garden-variety tiredness that a good night's sleep can fix. It is a profound, all-encompassing weariness. Even minor activities like climbing a single flight of stairs can leave you feeling completely drained, as if you have just run a marathon. Your muscles feel heavy, and your body is constantly craving rest. It is like your energy bank account is perpetually overdrawn. No matter how much you try to "deposit" with rest or relaxation, it is never enough to cover the "withdrawals" demanded by your daily activities.

Because this type of exhaustion does not fade, it significantly impacts your quality of life. Tasks that were once routine—like grocery shopping, cooking, or even socializing—become daunting challenges. It is not just physical; this constant fatigue can also wear down your mental and emotional resilience, making it harder to stay positive and motivated.

Slow Walking Speed: The Telltale Sign

Think back to those times when you were the leader of the pack during your morning walks, effortlessly outpacing everyone around you. But now, you might notice that others are speeding past, and you are struggling to keep up. That slower pace is not just about moving more leisurely; it can be an important sign of something more. Your muscles are the engines that power your movement. When they start to lose strength, it takes more effort to walk, making your once-brisk pace feel like a distant memory. Weak muscles mean you cannot push off the ground with the same force, causing each step to take a bit longer. Walking is not just about strong muscles; it also requires good balance and coordination. As these abilities decline, your steps may become shorter and slower. You might find yourself being extra cautious, taking smaller steps to avoid stumbling or falling. What used to be a quick jaunt around the block can now feel like an exhausting marathon. Slow walking speed means that your body is working much harder to cover the same distance. This increased effort can make you feel fatigued and can discourage you from staying active.

Walking speed is such a powerful indicator that it is often used in medical assessments. It can signal not just physical frailty, but also other underlying health issues. Researchers have found that slower walking speeds are linked to higher risks of disability and even shorter lifespans (81).

Low Physical Activity: The Sneaky Cycle of Decline

Remember when a morning jog was your go-to exercise? If that has now been replaced by a gentle stroll, it is not just a change in pace; it is a significant shift in your activity level. This transition can be a signal that your body is not as capable of handling vigorous activities as it once was. When you reduce your physical activity, it is often because your body is sending you signals. You might feel more tired, have less endurance, or find that your muscles and joints ache more after exercise. These signs suggest that your body is struggling to keep up with the demands of higher-intensity activities. Here is where it gets tricky: low physical activity can lead to more frailty, which in turn leads to even less activity. It is a downward spiral.

By keeping an eye on these physical markers, you can take proactive steps to maintain your strength and vitality. Whether it is through regular exercise, a balanced diet, or seeking medical advice, there are ways to combat the effects of frailty and continue living an active and fulfilling life. Remember, it is never too late to start taking care of yourself and investing in your health.

7.2 Cognitive And Emotional Aspects

Frailty is not just about the body—it is a full-body experience that includes the brain and emotions. Picture your mind as a busy office. With frailty, it is like the power goes out: the lights flicker, things slow down, and even simple tasks feel like climbing a mountain.

Memory Lane Detours

Frailty can play hide-and-seek with your memory. Names, dates, or that item you just added to your shopping list—poof, gone! While occasional forgetfulness happens to everyone (where did you leave your keys?), frailty-related cognitive changes can feel like your brain is running on low battery.

Imagine this: You are in the middle of a conversation, and suddenly you cannot recall the name of that actor from your favorite movie. It is frustrating, isn't it? Now, multiply that frustration by ten, and you will get an idea of what frailty-induced cognitive decline feels like. It is like having a mental traffic jam where thoughts and memories are bumper-to-bumper with no clear route to follow.

Memory problems associated with frailty can range from mild forgetfulness to more severe impairments that interfere with daily activities. It is not just about losing keys or forgetting names—it is about struggling to follow conversations, remember appointments, or even recognize familiar faces. These memory lapses can make everyday life want to navigate a maze with no map.

The good news? There are ways to combat this. Engaging in mentally stimulating activities like puzzles, reading, or even learning a new hobby can help keep your brain active. Just like you would exercise your muscles to keep them strong, exercising your brain can help maintain its function. Memory aids, such as using calendars, setting reminders, and keeping lists, can also be invaluable tools to manage cognitive challenges.

Mood Swings and Emotional Fog

Frailty can also mess with your emotional weather. You might feel like a storm cloud is following you around, with irritability, anxiety, or sadness rolling in out of nowhere. These emotional shifts are not just side effects; they are part of the package frailty brings, often linked to feeling less independent or capable.

Let us be real: nobody likes feeling like they have lost control over their lives. Frailty can lead to a loss of confidence and a sense of helplessness, which can trigger emotional responses. Imagine trying to bake a cake and suddenly finding that half the ingredients are missing—it is frustrating and disheartening. That is how frailty can make you feel about your abilities.

Mood swings can range from mild irritability to significant emotional distress. You might find yourself snapping at loved ones over minor inconveniences or feeling overwhelmed by simple tasks. Anxiety can creep in, making you worry about your health, your future, or your ability to handle daily activities. Depression might take hold, casting a shadow over your days and sapping your motivation.

But here is the silver lining: acknowledging these feelings and cognitive hiccups is the first step toward addressing them. Do not hesitate to bring in support—family, friends, or professionals who can offer solutions. Mindfulness exercises, such as meditation or deep-breathing techniques, can help manage stress and improve emotional well-being. Cognitive-behavioral therapy (CBT) can also be effective in addressing negative thought patterns and building resilience.

Staying socially active is another important strategy. Engaging with friends and family, participating in community activities, or joining support groups can provide emotional support and reduce feelings of isolation. Social interactions can boost your mood, provide a sense of belonging, and remind you that you are not alone in your journey. Remember, it is okay to seek help and use available resources to manage the cognitive and emotional aspects of frailty. Taking proactive steps can improve your quality of life, helping you navigate the challenges with greater ease and confidence.

7.3 How To Talk To Your Doctor About Frailty

Talking to your doctor about frailty might want to open up about a secret you did not want anyone to know. But here is the thing—your doctor is like a detective, and you are the key witness. Sharing your symptoms helps them solve the case of "Why am I feeling this way?"

Breaking the Ice

Starting the conversation about frailty can be daunting, but it does not have to be.

Think of it as catching up with an old friend. Start simple with something like, "I've noticed I'm feeling weaker lately," or "I'm losing weight and don't know why." Keep it conversational and straightforward. You do not need a PowerPoint presentation; just be honest about what is changed and how it is affecting your day-to-day life.

Consider framing it in everyday terms: "Doctor, I've been feeling like a balloon that's slowly losing air—my energy levels are just not what they used to be." This relatable analogy can help your doctor understand what you are going through without the need for medical jargon. Remember, your doctor is there to help you, and open communication is key to finding the best solutions.

Details, Details, Details

Doctors love specifics. They are like private detective piecing together a mystery, and every detail you provide is a vital clue. Mention things like, "I can't walk as far as I used to," or "I get tired halfway through doing the dishes." If it helps, jot down notes before your appointment. Write down what you have been experiencing, how long it has been happening, and any other changes you have noticed.

Think of it as preparing for a school report—only this time, you are reporting on your health. Specific examples like "I struggle to lift my grocery bags" or "I need to rest after climbing a flight of stairs" can paint a clear picture for your doctor. These details help your doctor understand the extent of your symptoms and guide them in finding the right tests or treatments for you.

Ask the Right Questions

Once you have laid it all out, turn the tables and ask questions of your own. Ask, "What could be causing this?" or "How can I stay stronger?" It is a two-way street, and you deserve answers that make sense. If your doctor uses terms, you do not understand, do not hesitate to ask for clarification. Say something like, "Can you explain that in simpler terms?" or "What does this mean for me?"

Additionally, asking about potential treatments and lifestyle changes can be incredibly helpful. Questions like, "What kind of exercises can I do to improve my strength?" or "Are there any dietary changes I should consider?" can provide you with actionable steps to take control of your health. Remember, your doctor is your ally in this journey, and their goal is to help you live your best life.

Follow-Up: The Sequel

Frailty is not a one-time chat; it is an ongoing conversation. Think of it as an epic TV series with multiple episodes. After your initial discussion, keep your doctor in the loop about new symptoms, what is working, and what is not. Regular follow-ups are essential to monitor your progress and make adjustments as needed.

Imagine your doctor as your co-pilot on this journey—they can help you navigate the turbulence and keep you flying steady. Schedule follow-up appointments to discuss how you are feeling and any changes you have noticed. Be proactive in sharing both the successes and the setbacks. If a particular treatment or exercise is not working, let your doctor know so they can suggest alternatives.

Remember, communication is key. Keeping an open line of dialogue with your doctor ensures that you are getting the best possible care. It also helps you stay informed and engaged in your health journey. Frailty is not the end of the road; it is just a detour. With awareness, action, and the right support, you can make it a smoother ride.

By recognizing these signs and symptoms and bringing them to the right people, you are taking the first step toward a healthier, more robust future. Frailty is a challenge, but with the right approach and a supportive healthcare team, you can manage its effects and maintain a good quality of life. So, do not be afraid to speak up and ask for the help you need—your health is worth it.

CHAPTER 8: UNDERSTANDING HEART DISEASE IN FRAIL ADULTS

Heart disease and frailty make quite a pair—a bit like the odd couple you never imagined, but somehow, they are always together at the party. In this chapter, we will delve into how heart disease presents differently in frail individuals, the challenges in diagnosis and treatment, and the special considerations for older adults. Get ready for a journey through the heart of this complex relationship.

8.1 How Heart Disease Presents Differently In Frail Adults

Picture this: heart disease in a young, spry adult might be like a car honking loudly at a green light—obvious and hard to ignore. But in frail individuals, it is more like a car with a subtle engine hiccup; the signs are there, but they are easy to miss.

For frail adults, the classic symptoms of heart disease—like chest pain and shortness of breath—can present quite differently (82). Imagine trying to spot a shy kitten in a room full of energetic puppies. In frail individuals, symptoms like fatigue, dizziness, and even unexplained weight loss might be the only clues. Instead of the dramatic chest-clutching scene you see in movies, you might notice your aunt is feeling unusually tired after her daily crossword puzzle.

Fatigue: The Stealthy Symptom

Fatigue in frail adults with heart disease (83, 84) is not just about feeling sleepy after a long day. It is like your phone battery draining faster than usual even after a full charge. They might struggle to find the energy to do simple tasks, like making breakfast or taking a short walk. This kind of fatigue can be a sneaky indicator that the heart is not pumping blood as efficiently as it should be.

Imagine waking up in the morning, expecting to feel refreshed and ready to tackle the day, only to realize your body feels like it has been through a marathon overnight. Frail adults might describe this fatigue as a constant, overwhelming tiredness that does not go away with rest. It is as if their internal energy meter is perpetually stuck on low. This type of fatigue can make everyday activities feel like to climb a steep hill. Tasks that once required little effort, like dressing or cooking, can become exhausting challenges. It is important to recognize that this fatigue is more than just a result of aging—it is a sign that the heart may be struggling to keep up with the body's demands.

Dizziness and Falls: The Unexpected Clues

Dizziness can often be overlooked or attributed to age. But in the context of frailty and heart disease, it is like a flashing warning light on your car's dashboard. Frail adults might experience frequent dizzy spells or even falls, which can be a sign of poor blood circulation due to heart problems (85). It is not just clumsiness; it is a clue that needs attention.

Imagine standing up after sitting for a while and feeling the room spin around you. For frail individuals, this dizzy sensation can occur more frequently and unpredictably. It is as if their body's internal balance system has gone haywire, making even simple movements feel unstable.

Frequent falls can be particularly dangerous for frail adults, leading to injuries that further complicate their health (85). If someone you know experiences frequent dizziness or falls, it is important to consider heart disease as a potential underlying cause. This symptom can indicate that the heart is not pumping enough blood to the brain, leading to moments of disorientation and imbalance.

Unexplained Weight Loss: The Hidden Signal

Unintentional weight loss in frail individuals can be a sign that the body is working extra hard to keep up with the demands of a struggling heart. It is like a bank account slowly draining without any big purchases—there is something going on behind the scenes. Noticing these subtle changes can be the first step in identifying heart disease in frail adults.

Imagine noticing that your favorite pair of pants, which used to fit perfectly, now hangs loosely on your waist. Unexplained weight loss might seem like a positive change at first, but for frail adults, it can be a red flag. When the heart struggles to pump efficiently, the body may start to break down muscle and fat to meet its energy needs. This weight loss is not due to dieting or increased physical activity; it is a result of the body's internal struggle to function properly. Frail adults might lose their appetite, leading to reduced food intake and further weight loss. It is important to monitor these changes and consult a healthcare professional if you notice significant, unexplained weight loss.

Beyond the Obvious: Subtle Clues to Watch For

In addition to these primary symptoms, there are other subtle clues of heart disease in frail individuals that often go unnoticed. These can include:

Swelling in the Legs and Ankles: Fluid retention can cause swelling, especially in the lower extremities. This can be a sign of heart failure, where the heart is not pumping blood effectively.

Shortness of Breath: While not as dramatic as the classic chest pain, shortness of breath can be a significant symptom. It might occur during physical activity or even when lying down.

Confusion and Memory Issues: Poor blood circulation can affect brain function, leading to cognitive changes such as confusion or memory problems.

Recognizing these indicators and understanding how heart disease presents differently in frail individuals is important for timely diagnosis and treatment. It is like putting together a puzzle—each piece of information helps create a clearer picture of the individual's health. By paying attention to these subtle changes and seeking medical advice, you can help ensure that frail adults receive the care they need to manage heart disease effectively. This proactive approach can significantly improve their quality of life and overall well-being.

8.2 Challenges In Diagnosis And Treatment

Diagnosing and treating heart disease in frail individuals (13) can feel like solving a particularly tricky puzzle. It is not just about finding the right piece; it is about understanding how each piece fits together in the bigger picture.

Diagnosing Heart Disease: The Puzzle Pieces

One of the biggest challenges in diagnosing heart disease in frail adults is that the symptoms can be masked by other conditions. It is like trying to hear a whisper in a noisy room. For instance, shortness of breath might be dismissed as a normal part of aging or a symptom of another illness. But when combined with other subtle signals like fatigue or dizziness, it can point to an underlying heart issue.

The Role of Comprehensive Assessments

To accurately diagnose heart disease in frail individuals, doctors often rely on comprehensive assessments (13). Think of it as a detective gathering clues from multiple sources. These assessments can include detailed medical histories, physical exams, blood tests, and imaging studies, past and present. The goal is to piece together all the information to form a clear picture of the patient's health.

Management Challenges: Balancing Act

Managing heart disease in frail adults requires a delicate balance. It is like walking a tightrope with a stack of plates. On one hand, you need to address the heart condition effectively; on the other, you must consider the individual's overall frailty and vulnerability. Medications that are effective in younger, healthier individuals might have different effects or side effects in frail adults.

Personalized Care Plans

Creating a personalized treatment plan is essential. This involves tailoring the approach to the individual's specific needs and conditions. It might include a combination of medications, lifestyle changes, and therapies designed to improve both heart health and overall well-being.

The key is to find a treatment regimen that works without causing additional harm or stress.

8.3 Special Considerations For Older Adults

Older adults have unique needs and considerations when it comes to heart disease and frailty (86). It is not just about adding more years to life; it is about adding more life to those years.

The Importance of Holistic Care

Holistic care for frail older adults with heart disease means looking beyond the heart (87). It is about considering the whole person, including their physical, emotional, and social well-being. Imagine it as tending to a garden; you do not just water one plant, you care for the entire ecosystem to ensure everything thrives.

Physical Activity: Finding the Right Balance

While exercise is beneficial, it is important to find the right balance for frail individuals. Think of it as tuning a musical instrument—you need just the right amount of tension to produce beautiful music. Low-impact activities like walking, swimming, or gentle yoga can help improve cardiovascular health without overexerting the body.

Nutrition: Fuel for the Journey

Proper nutrition plays a vital role in managing both heart disease and frailty. A balanced diet rich in fruits, vegetables, whole grains, and lean proteins can provide the necessary nutrients to support heart health and overall vitality. Consulting with a nutritionist can help create a tailored plan that meets individual needs.

Mental and Emotional Well-being

Addressing the mental and emotional aspects of health is equally important. Frail older adults with heart disease may experience anxiety, depression, or feelings of isolation. Providing support through counseling, social activities, and community resources can help improve their quality of life. It is like adding sunshine to a garden—nurturing the mind and spirit is essential for overall well-being.

Regular Check-Ups: Staying on Course

Regular medical check-ups are necessary for monitoring the health of frail older adults with heart disease. Think of it as keeping your car in good shape with regular maintenance. These check-ups allow for early detection of any changes or complications, ensuring that the treatment plan remains effective, and adjustments can be made as needed.

By understanding the unique challenges and considerations for older adults with heart disease and frailty, we can provide better care and support for a healthier future. It is about creating a comprehensive approach that addresses all aspects of health and well-being, helping individuals live their best lives despite the challenges they face.

Now that you have delved into the specifics of how heart disease affects frail adults, it becomes clear that this relationship is complicated and multifaceted. Yet, with the right knowledge and proactive care, managing these conditions is not only possible but can lead to a significantly improved quality of life for those affected. Here is to a healthier, more informed future!

CHAPTER 9: FRAILTY IN HEART FAILURE

Frailty and heart disease go together like peanut butter and jelly—only a lot less tasty and a lot more complicated. In this chapter, we will delve into why frailty is so common in advanced heart failure and other heart diseases, how to manage symptoms while improving quality of life, and the crucial role of rehabilitative care. Buckle up for a heart-to-heart on managing these intertwined conditions.

9.1 Why Frailty Is Common In Heart Failure

Frailty often tags along with advanced heart failure and other chronic heart diseases (88) like an unwelcome guest who never leaves. But why is this connection so strong? Let us break it down in simple terms.

The Energy Drain

Picture your heart as the engine of a car. In heart failure, this engine starts sputtering—it cannot pump blood efficiently, leading to less oxygen and nutrients being delivered to your muscles and organs. It is like trying to drive up a steep hill with a lawnmower engine. This inefficiency drains your energy, making you feel weak and tired—classic signals of frailty.

Think of it this way: your body is constantly demanding fuel (oxygen and nutrients), but your heart is like a tiny, tired engine that cannot keep up with the demand. This lack of efficient blood flow results in muscle weakness and overall fatigue. It is not just a bad day—it is your heart struggling to keep everything running smoothly. Over time, this persistent energy drain can lead to a downward spiral of weakness and frailty.

The Inactivity Loop

Heart disease can create a vicious cycle of inactivity (89). When your heart struggles, everyday activities like walking to the mailbox or climbing stairs can leave you breathless. Because these tasks become harder, you might start avoiding them, leading to decreased physical activity. This inactivity further weakens your muscles and reduces your endurance, deepening the cycle of frailty.

Imagine you are trying to stay active, but every step feels like trudging through thick mud. The effort required to move around becomes so overwhelming that it is easier to just sit down and rest. But the more you rest, the weaker your muscles become. It is like a snowball effect—less activity leads to more weakness, making it even harder to stay active. Breaking this cycle requires a carefully balanced approach to exercise and rest.

Malnutrition and Weight Loss

Heart disease can also mess with your appetite. When your heart's not working properly, your body's metabolism can go haywire. You might lose your appetite or have difficulty eating, leading to weight loss. This unintended weight loss often means you are losing muscle mass too, further contributing to frailty.

Think of your body as a finely tuned machine that needs the right fuel to function. When heart disease interferes with your ability to eat properly, it is like running a car on empty. Your body starts to cannibalize its own muscle tissue for energy, leading to a decrease in strength and endurance. This weight loss is not the kind you celebrate—it is a sign that your body is struggling to cope with the demands placed on it by heart disease.

Hormonal Changes

Advanced heart failure can trigger hormonal imbalances. Stress hormones like adrenaline and cortisol can be elevated, and these hormonal changes can break down muscle tissue and promote inflammation. It is like your body's alarm system is stuck in overdrive, wearing you down over time.

Imagine your body is constantly on high alert, as if you are preparing for an emergency that never ends. These elevated stress hormones wreak havoc on your muscles, breaking them down and making it harder for your body to repair itself. This chronic state of stress can lead to further weakening of your muscles and contribute to the overall frailty associated with advanced heart failure.

The Impact of Chronic Inflammation

Like any other heart disease, heart failure and frailty can also be linked through chronic inflammation. When the heart is under constant strain, it can lead to an inflammatory response throughout the body. This inflammation can damage tissues and organs, including muscles, leading to weakness and fatigue.

Picture inflammation as a fire smouldering inside your body. It is not the raging kind that demands immediate attention, but rather a slow burn that steadily causes damage over time. This chronic inflammation can exacerbate frailty by further weakening the muscles and other vital tissues, making it even harder for individuals to maintain their strength and function.

Understanding these connections helps in recognizing why frailty is so prevalent among individuals with advanced heart failure and other chronic heart diseases. It sets the stage for addressing these challenges head-on. By acknowledging the linkages, we can develop better strategies to manage both heart failure and frailty, improving the overall quality of life for those affected. The goal is to break the cycle of frailty by addressing these underlying causes, helping individuals maintain their strength and vitality despite the challenges posed by heart failure. It is about finding a balance and taking proactive steps to ensure that frailty does not overshadow the lives of those dealing with heart failure.

9.2 Managing Symptoms And Improving Quality Of Life

Managing symptoms and improving quality of life in frail individuals with heart failure is like fine-tuning a delicate machine. It requires attention to detail, patience, and a holistic approach.

Symptom Management: The Balancing Act

Effective symptom management starts with a clear plan. Medications play a crucial role in managing heart failure symptoms, but they must be carefully balanced to avoid side effects that can exacerbate frailty. Diuretics, for instance, help reduce fluid buildup but can cause dehydration if not monitored properly.

Regular check-ups are essential. Think of them as pit stops in a long race—they allow your healthcare team to adjust medications, check for new symptoms, and ensure you are on the right track. Keeping a symptom diary can also be helpful. Note down how you are feeling each day, any new symptoms, and how you are responding to treatments. This diary becomes a valuable tool for your doctor to fine-tune your care plan.

Nutrition: The Fuel You Need

Good nutrition is the backbone of managing frailty in heart failure. Imagine your body as a garden; it needs the right nutrients to thrive. A balanced diet rich in fruits, vegetables, whole grains, and lean proteins can provide the fuel your body needs to maintain strength and energy. Consider consulting with a nutritionist who can tailor a diet plan to your specific needs. They can help you find foods that are not only nutritious but also easy to eat, especially if you have a decreased appetite. Small, frequent meals might be more manageable than three large ones, ensuring you get enough calories and nutrients throughout the day.

Physical Activity: Staying Active Safely

Staying active is crucial, but it must be done safely. Think of exercise as oiling the gears of a machine; it keeps everything running smoothly. Low-impact activities like walking, jogging, swimming, or yoga can help maintain muscle strength and improve cardiovascular health without overexerting your body.

Working with a physical therapist can be beneficial. They can design an exercise program tailored to your abilities and needs, ensuring you stay active without risking injury. Even small activities, like gentle stretching or light resistance exercises, can make a big difference in maintaining mobility and strength.

Emotional and Mental Health: The Hidden Elements

Do not overlook the emotional and mental aspects of managing frailty and heart failure. It is like maintaining the software of a computer—essential for overall function. Stress, anxiety, and depression can all impact your physical health. Seeking support through counseling, support groups, or stress-reducing practices like prayers, meditation and mindfulness can improve your overall well-being. By addressing these different elements, you can manage symptoms more effectively and improve your quality of life, even in the presence of frailty and heart disease.

9.3 Role Of Rehabilitative Care

Rehabilitative care is a game-changer for individuals dealing with frailty and heart failure (76). It is like having a team of experts fine-tune your body and mind, helping you get back to living your best life.

Cardiac Rehabilitation: A Lifeline

Cardiac rehabilitation programs are designed specifically for individuals with heart disease (77). These programs combine exercise training, education on heart-healthy living, and counseling to reduce stress. Imagine it as boot camp for your heart—intensive but incredibly beneficial.

Through supervised exercise sessions, you will learn how to exercise safely and effectively. The goal is to improve your cardiovascular fitness, strengthen your muscles, and boost your overall energy levels. Education sessions cover topics like nutrition, medication management, and lifestyle changes, empowering you with the knowledge to take control of your health.

Physical Therapy: Moving with Confidence

Physical therapy focuses on improving your strength, mobility, and balance. Think of your physical therapist as a personal coach, guiding you through exercises that enhance your physical capabilities without overexerting you. They can help you develop strategies to manage daily activities more easily, reducing the risk of falls and other injuries. A tailored physical therapy program can address specific issues related to frailty, such as muscle weakness and joint stiffness. By working closely with your physical therapist, you can build confidence in your movements and improve your overall physical function.

Occupational Therapy: Enhancing Daily Living

Occupational therapy helps you maintain your independence by focusing on the skills you need for daily living. Imagine an occupational therapist as a problem-solver, helping you find ways to perform everyday tasks more easily and safely. They can recommend assistive devices, like grab bars or shower chairs, to make your home environment safer. They can also teach you techniques to conserve energy, such as breaking tasks into smaller steps and using proper body mechanics. By addressing these practical aspects of daily living, occupational therapy helps you maintain your independence and improve your quality of life.

Support Networks: Building a Community

Finally, building a strong support network is crucial. This network can include family, friends, healthcare providers, and support groups. Think of it as assembling a team of cheerleaders who are there to support you every step of the way. Support groups, whether in-person or online, provide a space to share experiences, gain new insights, and find emotional support from others who understand what you are going through. Regular interactions with your support network can boost your morale and provide practical advice for managing frailty and heart disease.

By embracing rehabilitative care, you can enhance your physical, emotional, and mental well-being, paving the way for a healthier future despite the challenges of frailty and heart failure. It is about taking proactive steps to live your best life, with the support and guidance of your healthcare team and loved ones.

CHAPTER 10: NUTRITION AND FRAILTY

10.1 Foods That Fight Frailty And Support Heart Health

When it comes to staying strong and keeping your heart happy, food is not just fuel—it is medicine. Picture your meals as little packages of power, brimming with nutrients that help your body fight frailty. But what does a frailty-fighting diet look like? Spoiler alert: It is not all kale and quinoa. Though already described in each chapter with relevant sections, let us dive into the review of the delicious world of heart-healthy foods that pack a punch against frailty (90).

Fruits and Vegetables: The Superheroes of Nutrition

Start with the basics: fruits and vegetables (91). These colorful delights are the superheroes of the food world. They are packed with antioxidants that protect your body from the wear and tear of aging. Think of them as tiny shields for your cells, blocking damage from the inside out. Leafy greens like spinach and broccoli are especially good for your heart and muscles.

Antioxidant Powerhouses

Berries, such as blueberries, strawberries, and raspberries, are bursting with antioxidants. These tiny fruits are like the secret agents of nutrition, stealthily combating free radicals and reducing inflammation. Incorporate a variety of fruits and veggies into your diet to ensure you are getting a wide range of nutrients. Aim for a rainbow on your plate—each color represents different vitamins and minerals that support overall health.

Whole Grains: The Sustaining Energy Providers

Whole grains are another MVP. Brown rice, oats, and whole-grain bread provide the energy your body needs to stay active and vibrant. Plus, they are great for heart health, keeping your blood sugar steady and your belly full. Think of whole grains as the slow-burning fuel that keeps your engine running smoothly throughout the day.

Fiber-Rich Choices

Whole grains are rich in dietary fiber, which aids in digestion and helps maintain a healthy weight. Fiber also plays a role in lowering cholesterol levels, further supporting heart health. Incorporate quinoa, barley, and whole-wheat pasta into your meals to enjoy their benefits. These grains are versatile and can be used in a variety of dishes, from salads to soups to main courses.

Healthy Fats: The Heart's Best Friends

Do not forget healthy fats! Yes, you heard that right—fat can be your friend. Avocados, nuts, seeds, and olive oil are rich in omega-3 fatty acids, which reduce inflammation and keep your heart ticking along smoothly. These fats are like the calm peacemakers in your body, reducing the chaos of inflammation and promoting overall health.

Omega-3 Fatty Acids

Fatty fish, such as salmon, mackerel, and sardines, are excellent sources of omega-3s. These fatty acids support heart health by reducing triglycerides, lowering blood pressure, and preventing the buildup of plaque in the arteries (92). Nuts and seeds, like walnuts and flaxseeds, are also great sources of omega-3s and can be easily added to salads, yogurts, or smoothies.

Lean Proteins: Building Blocks of Strength

Then there is the protein. We will dive deeper into this in the next section, but here is the gist: lean proteins like chicken, fish, beans, and tofu are the building blocks of your muscles. And strong muscles mean a more robust, less frail you. Protein is like the construction crew for your body, constantly repairing and building your strength.

Plant-Based Proteins

Beans, lentils, and chickpeas are not only rich in protein but also packed with fiber and essential nutrients. These plant-based proteins are versatile and can be used in a variety of dishes, from soups and stews to salads and dips. Tofu and tempeh are excellent alternatives for those looking to reduce their intake of animal products, providing high-quality protein without the saturated fats found in some meats.

Hydration: The Unsung Hero

Lastly, let us give a shoutout to hydration. Water does not get the credit it deserves, but staying hydrated keeps everything in your body working better, from your joints to your digestion. Plus, dehydration can mimic frailty symptoms, like weakness and dizziness—so drink up! Water is the silent hero.

Creative Hydration Solutions

To make hydration more enjoyable, try infusing your water with slices of cucumber, lemon, or berries. Herbal teas and broths are also excellent options to keep you hydrated. Remember, hydration is not just about drinking water—foods with high water content, like watermelon, cucumbers, and oranges, also contribute to your overall fluid intake.

Making It Practical and Delicious

Incorporating these foods into your daily diet does not have to be a chore. Here are some tips to make eating healthy enjoyable and practical:

Meal Prep: Prepare and portion out your meals in advance to save time and ensure you have healthy options readily available.

Mix and Match: Combine different fruits, veggies, whole grains, proteins, and healthy fats to create diverse and delicious meals.

Experiment: Do not be afraid to try new recipes and ingredients. Cooking can be a fun and creative way to explore new flavors and cuisines.

Snack Smart: Keep healthy snacks like nuts, yogurt, and fruit on hand for quick and nutritious bites.

By focusing on these nutrient-rich foods, you can create a diet that not only fights frailty but also supports your heart health. It is about making mindful choices that nourish your body and enhance your quality of life. So, let us toast to eating well and living strong—cheers with a glass of water, of course!

10.2 The Role Of Protein And Micronutrients

If your body were a car, protein would be the steel keeping it sturdy, while micronutrients would be the nuts and bolts holding it all together. Without enough of these essential nutrients, the machine starts to wobble—and no one wants that. So, let us dive into why protein and micronutrients are crucial in the battle against frailty and how they support heart health (93).

Protein: The Body's Repair Crew

Protein is the star player here. Think of it as the repair crew for your body. Every time you lift a grocery bag, climb stairs, or even smile, your muscles use protein to rebuild and grow stronger. And as you age, your protein needs go up, not down. That is because your muscles naturally shrink over time—a sneaky condition called sarcopenia. To fight back, aim for a palm-sized portion of protein at every meal.

Sources of Protein

Eggs, fish, poultry, beans, and dairy are all excellent sources of protein. Do not like cooking? Grab a handful of nuts or a cup of Greek yogurt. Prefer plant-based? Tofu, lentils, and chickpeas have your back. Here is a quick rundown of protein-rich foods to include in your diet:

Eggs: Versatile and easy to prepare, eggs are a great way to start your day with a protein boost.

Fish: Salmon, tuna, and other fatty fish are rich in protein and omega-3 fatty acids, which support heart health.

Poultry: Chicken and turkey are lean sources of protein that can be used in a variety of dishes.

Beans and Legumes: Black beans, lentils, and chickpeas are not only rich in protein but also packed with fiber and essential nutrients.

Dairy: Milk, cheese, and yogurt provide high-quality protein along with calcium and vitamin D.

Nuts and Seeds: Almonds, walnuts, and chia seeds make for nutritious snacks that are high in protein and healthy fats.

Protein is like the construction crew for your body, constantly repairing and building your strength. By incorporating a variety of protein sources into your diet, you can ensure that your muscles have the fuel they need to stay strong and healthy.

Micronutrients: The Little Guys with Big Jobs

Now, onto micronutrients—the little guys with big jobs. These vitamins and minerals might be tiny, but they are mighty when it comes to maintaining your health and fighting frailty.

Calcium and Vitamin D: The Bone Builders

Calcium and vitamin D are crucial for bone health, which is a key part of staying mobile and independent. Foods like milk, cheese, yogurt, and fortified cereals are great sources. Not a fan of dairy? Try leafy greens or almond milk. Calcium supports bone strength, while vitamin D helps your body absorb calcium more effectively.

Calcium Sources: Dairy products, leafy greens (like kale and broccoli), almonds, and fortified plant-based milks.

Vitamin D Sources: Sunlight exposure, fatty fish, fortified dairy products, and supplements if needed.

Imagine these nutrients as the architects and builders of your bones, ensuring they remain strong and resilient.

Iron: The Energizer

Iron is another biggie, especially if you feel tired all the time. It helps your blood carry oxygen to your muscles, keeping you energized. Red meat, spinach, and legumes are your iron-rich friends. Pair them with vitamin C (like an orange) to help your body absorb the iron better.

Iron Sources: Red meat, poultry, seafood, beans, spinach, and fortified cereals.

Vitamin C Sources: Citrus fruits (oranges, lemons), bell peppers, strawberries, and tomatoes.

Think of iron as the fuel that powers your body's engine, keeping you active and alert.

B Vitamins: The Brain Boosters

Let us not forget the B vitamins, which keep your energy levels up and your brain sharp. Whole grains, fish, and eggs are packed with these mental boosters. B vitamins (such as B6, B12, and folate) support brain function, nerve health, and energy metabolism.

B Vitamin Sources: Whole grains (brown rice, oatmeal), fish (salmon, trout), eggs, legumes, and leafy greens.

These vitamins are like the electrical wiring in your body, ensuring everything runs smoothly and efficiently.

Zinc: The Immune Supporter

Zinc, found in seafood and seeds, also plays a role in keeping your immune system humming along. It is crucial for wound healing, immune function, and protein synthesis.

Zinc Sources: Seafood (oysters, crab), poultry, beans, nuts, and seeds (pumpkin seeds, sesame seeds).

Imagine zinc as the security system for your body, protecting you from invaders and helping you recover from illnesses.

Putting It All Together: A Nutrient-Rich Diet

To fight frailty and support heart health, it is essential to include a variety of protein sources and micronutrient-rich foods in your diet (93). Here are some practical tips to make it easier:

Diversify Your Plate: Aim to include different protein sources and micronutrients in every meal. Mix and match foods to keep your meals interesting and nutritious.

Snack Smartly: Keep healthy snacks like nuts, yogurt, and fruit on hand for a quick and nutritious energy boost.

Stay Hydrated: Drink plenty of water throughout the day. Hydration supports overall health and can prevent symptoms of frailty.

Consult a Nutritionist: If you are unsure about your nutrient intake, a nutritionist can help you create a personalized diet plan that meets your specific needs.

By focusing on the role of protein and micronutrients, you can build a strong foundation for your health, keeping frailty at bay and supporting a healthy heart. Remember, it is all about balance and making mindful choices that nourish your body and enhance your well-being. So, let us eat well, live strong, and enjoy the journey to better health!

10.3 Practical Tips For Frail Adults

Eating well does not have to be complicated or boring. In fact, it can—and should—be delicious! Here are some simple, practical tips to make frailty-fighting meals a breeze:

Stock Up on Staples

Keep your kitchen filled with easy-to-use basics like canned beans, frozen veggies, and whole-grain pasta. These are lifesavers on busy or low-energy days. Having these staples on hand ensures that you can whip up a nutritious meal even when you are not feeling your best. Think of your pantry as your personal mini-mart, stocked with all the essentials to keep you going.

Canned Beans: These are a quick source of protein and fiber. Add them to salads, soups, or stews for an instant nutrient boost.

Frozen Vegetables: Equally nutritious as fresh ones, frozen veggies are a convenient option for adding vitamins and minerals to your meals. Plus, they have a long shelf life, so you always have veggies on hand, if you don't access to the fresh ones.

Whole-Grain Pasta: Whole grains provide sustained energy and keep your blood sugar stable. Pair pasta with a simple tomato sauce and some veggies for a quick, balanced meal.

Go for Mini-Meals

If you find big meals overwhelming, break your day into smaller, snack-sized portions. A boiled egg and a slice of whole-grain toast, a handful of almonds with a banana, or a small bowl of lentil soup can pack a nutritious punch without overwhelming your appetite. Think of these mini-meals as constant little energy boosts throughout the day.

Breakfast: Start with a boiled egg and a piece of whole-grain toast. It is a simple, protein-rich meal to kickstart your morning.

Mid-Morning Snack: A handful of almonds paired with a banana provides a perfect blend of protein, healthy fats, and carbs to keep you going.

Lunch: A small bowl of lentil soup is hearty and full of fiber and protein, making it a filling yet light meal.

Dinner: For dinner, enjoy a serving of grilled salmon accompanied by a side of steamed vegetables and quinoa. The salmon provides heart-healthy omega-3 fatty acids, the veggies add essential vitamins and minerals, and the quinoa offers a good source of protein and fiber to complete your nutritious day.

Sneak in Nutrition

Add spinach to your morning smoothie, sprinkle seeds on your cereal, or mix powdered protein into your oatmeal. Small tweaks can make a big difference. Think of this as ninja nutrition—sneaking in extra nutrients without much effort.

Morning Smoothie: Add a handful of spinach to your favorite fruit smoothie. It boosts your intake of vitamins and minerals without altering the taste significantly.

Breakfast Cereal: Sprinkle chia seeds or flaxseeds on top for added omega-3 fatty acids and fiber.

Oatmeal: Mix in a scoop of protein powder to increase the protein content and keep you feeling full longer.

Cook Once, Eat Twice

Batch cooking is your friend. Make a big pot of chicken soup or a veggie-packed casserole, then freeze portions for later. It is like giving your future self a healthy gift. This method saves time and ensures you always have a homemade meal ready to go.

Chicken Soup: A large pot of chicken soup can be portioned into individual servings and frozen. Just reheat and enjoy for an easy, nutritious meal.

Veggie Casserole: Pack it full of your favorite vegetables, cook, and then freeze in portions. It is a versatile dish that you can enjoy multiple times.

Get Creative with Drinks

Struggling to chew? Try nutrient-rich drinks like smoothies or protein shakes. Drinks can be a great way to get nutrients without the need to chew.

Smoothies: Blend together milk, a banana, spinach, and peanut butter for a creamy, nutrient-packed drink.

Protein Shakes: Add protein powder to your preferred milk or milk alternative, along with some fruit and greens, for a quick and easy meal.

Make It Social

Share meals with friends or family whenever you can. Not only is this great for your mental health, but it also makes eating more enjoyable. Food is meant to be shared, and dining with others can make meals more enjoyable and less of a chore.

Family Dinners: Invite family members over for a weekly meal. It is a great way to stay connected and enjoy a home-cooked meal together.

Potluck Gatherings: Organize a potluck with friends where everyone brings a dish. This not only reduces the cooking burden but also introduces you to new dishes and recipes.

Ask for Help

If shopping or cooking feels overwhelming, do not hesitate to ask for help. Whether it is a meal delivery service, a family member, or a community group, there is no shame in getting a little support. Remember, asking for help is a strength, not a weakness.

Meal Delivery Services: There are many services that deliver healthy, pre-made meals to your door. This can be a great option if you are struggling to cook.

Family and Friends: Do not be afraid to ask loved ones for help with grocery shopping or meal prep. They are often more than happy to lend a hand.

Community Groups: Look into local community groups or senior centers that offer meal programs or assistance.

Stay Inspired and Enjoy the Process

Remember, every bite counts. By choosing nourishing foods and making eating an enjoyable part of your day, you are not just filling your stomach—you are fuelling your future. And that is something to toast to (with a green smoothie, of course)! Keep experimenting with new recipes, involve loved ones in meal preparation, and most importantly, enjoy the process. Eating well is a journey, and with these practical tips, you can make it a delicious and fulfilling one.

CHAPTER 11: EXERCISE AND FRAILTY

If exercise came in a pill, it would be the most prescribed drug in the world. But here is the good news: you do not need a prescription to get started! Exercise is your body's best defense against frailty and a key to keeping your heart and body strong (61). It is like upgrading your engine while you are driving—practical, effective, and surprisingly doable. This chapter explores how movement can be transformative, especially for older adults dealing with frailty and heart disease. Whether you are taking your first cautious steps or looking to regain lost stamina, there is something here for everyone.

11.1 Safe Exercises For The Frail Heart

When it comes to starting an exercise routine with a frail heart, it is perfectly normal to feel hesitant. After all, you want to build strength, not stress. But here is the truth: moving your body—even gently—can work wonders. Safe does not have to mean boring, and every little step (or stretch) can add up to big improvements in your heart health and overall well-being.

Start with the Basics: Movement is Medicine

Think of your body like a classic car—it runs better when you take it out for a spin, even if it is just around the block. Movement helps keep your joints flexible, your muscles engaged, and your blood flowing smoothly. And the best part? You do not need to start with a marathon.

Begin with small, manageable activities. A 10-minute stroll around your living room, a few toe taps while seated, or even some gentle stretches can make a difference. These might seem tiny, but they are like planting seeds for a healthier you. Over time, they will grow into stronger muscles, better balance, and a happier heart.

Chair Exercises: Your New Best Friend

If walking feels intimidating, pull up a chair—literally! Chair exercises are a fantastic way to ease into movement. Start with seated marches to get your legs moving or try leg lifts to strengthen your lower body. Want to work your arms? Use soup cans for some gentle bicep curls. Bonus: you can do all this while catching up on your favorite TV shows!

Stretches: Simple Yet Effective

Stretching is like a wake-up call for your body. Gentle stretches help improve your flexibility and circulation without putting too much strain on your heart. Reach for the sky, twist gently from side to side, or try touching your toes (or your knees—no pressure!).

Get the Green Light

Before you jump into any exercise routine, it is important to get your doctor's approval. Think of them as your heart's personal trainer—they know what is safe and what is not. Whether it is a brisk walk, some light yoga, or splashing around in a pool, your doctor can help tailor a plan that fits your specific needs.

Why the Green Light Matters

Your heart is a hardworking organ, and it deserves a plan designed just for it. Getting medical advice ensures that you are exercising within a safe range for your condition. Plus, it is a chance to discuss any concerns you might have, like shortness of breath or fatigue.

Low-Impact Favorites

Doctors often recommend low-impact activities for people with frail hearts. Walking is a classic choice—it is free, simple, and effective. Water aerobics is another gem; the buoyancy of water reduces stress on your joints while giving your heart a gentle workout. And do not underestimate yoga! Its combination of stretching and deep breathing can be incredibly calming and heart-friendly.

Make it Fun

Let us be real: the word "exercise" does not always scream excitement. But who says workouts have to be dull? The secret to sticking with it is to make it enjoyable.

Dance Like Nobody's Watching

Turn up your favorite tunes and let loose in your living room. Whether it is a slow waltz or a shimmy to your go-to pop hits, dancing is a fantastic way to get moving and have fun. Plus, it is good for your heart—and your soul!

Buddy Up

Everything is better with a friend. Invite a neighbour for a walk, join a group class, or simply FaceTime a friend while you exercise. The social connection is a heart booster in itself, and having a companion makes it more likely you will stick with your routine.

Gamify It

Set small, playful goals to keep yourself motivated. Maybe it is walking to the end of the driveway without stopping or doing 10 chair squats during commercial breaks. Celebrate each victory—you are winning at life!

The Rule of Progress

Rome was not built in a day, and neither is a fitter, stronger you. The key to success is starting small and building up gradually. This is not a race—it is a journey, and every step counts.

Baby Steps, Big Rewards

Cannot walk for more than five minutes? That is okay! Start with what you can do. If you manage five minutes today, aim for six tomorrow. Over time, those small increases will add up to significant gains.

Listen to Your Body

Progress does not mean pushing through pain. If something does not feel right, stop, and reassess. Your body knows what it needs, so give it the respect it deserves. And do not beat yourself up if you need a rest day—it is part of the process.

Track Your Wins

Keep a journal of your progress. Write down how far you walked, how many stretches you did, or how you felt afterward. It is incredibly motivating to look back and see how far you have come.

To recap, safe exercises for the frail heart are all about building confidence and strength without overdoing it. Start small, keep it fun, and celebrate your progress. Remember, every little bit of movement helps, and with time and consistency, you will feel the difference in your heart, muscles, and overall well-being. So, take that first step—you have got this!

11.2 Building Strength And Stamina

Strength and stamina are not just for marathon runners or gym enthusiasts—they are for anyone who wants to make everyday life easier and more enjoyable. Whether it is carrying groceries, playing with your grandkids, or walking up a flight of stairs without gasping for air, building strength and stamina can help you reclaim your independence and confidence. Think of strength training and endurance exercises as your personal Avengers team. They work together to tackle frailty and keep your body resilient. No spandex required, though—you can start small, right in the comfort of your home.

Muscles Are Your Body's Best Friends

Let us talk muscles. These bundles of power do more than look good in a tank top. Strong muscles support your bones, improve your balance, and make life's little tasks—like opening jars or getting out of a chair—a lot easier. Plus, they are great allies for your heart, helping it work more efficiently. Here is the best part: you do not need a gym membership or fancy equipment to start building muscle. In fact, your pantry might hold everything you need!

Soup Cans for Biceps: If you don't have access to regular gym instruments, don't be disheartened. Grab two cans of soup (or any similar-sized items) and do some bicep curls. It is strength training with a side of dinner prep.

Chair Squats: Stand up and sit down from a chair without using your hands. It sounds simple, but it is a sneaky way to strengthen your legs and core.

Wall Push-Ups: Regular push-ups might feel intimidating, but wall push-ups are their gentler cousin. Stand a few steps away from a wall, place your hands on it, and push in and out. It is easy on the joints but tough on your muscles.

Remember, even superheroes had to start somewhere. If your muscles feel a little wobbly at first, that is a good sign—they are waking up and getting stronger!

The Power of Endurance

Strength is only half the story. Stamina—or endurance—is what keeps you going. It is the ability to do activities for longer periods without feeling like you have just run a marathon (unless you actually are running a marathon, in which case, hats off to you!). Endurance exercises are great for your heart and lungs, helping them work more efficiently. They also boost your energy levels and can even lift your mood. Here is how to get started:

Walking Wonders: A brisk walk is one of the simplest and most effective ways to build stamina. Start with five minutes and add a minute each day. Before you know it, you will be strolling like a pro.

Pedal Power: A stationary bike is a great option if walking feels too hard on your joints. You can cycle while watching your favorite TV show—it is multitasking at its healthiest.

Gardening Glory: Yes, gardening counts as exercise! Digging, planting, and weeding get your heart pumping and your muscles working. Plus, you get a beautiful garden as a bonus.

Here is a secret: consistency beats intensity every time. You do not need to go all out; you just need to keep showing up. Think of it like saving money—small deposits add up over time.

Rest and Recovery: The Unsung Heroes

Here is something most people do not realize: rest days are just as important as workout days. When you exercise, you are essentially breaking your muscles down. It is during rest that they repair themselves and grow stronger. So, if you are sore or tired, listen to your body—it is asking for a timeout. Recovery does not have to mean doing nothing. Gentle activities like stretching, yoga, or a leisurely walk can help ease stiffness and keep your body in motion without overdoing it.

Also, do not underestimate the power of sleep. Quality sleep gives your body the time it needs to repair and recharge. Think of it as plugging your phone into the charger overnight —essential for optimal performance the next day. If you feel guilty about resting, here is a comforting thought: even professional athletes have rest days, and they are doing just fine.

Small Wins Lead to Big Changes

The journey to building strength and stamina is all about baby steps. You do not need to transform into a fitness guru overnight. Celebrate the small victories, whether it is walking an extra block, lifting a heavier can, or simply feeling less tired after a day's activities. And remember, exercise is not just about adding years to your life—it is about adding life to your years. With stronger muscles and better stamina, you will not only feel more capable but also more confident in tackling whatever life throws your way. So, grab those soup cans, lace up your sneakers, and let us get moving. Your future self will thank you!

11.3 Role Of Cardiac Rehabilitation

Imagine your heart as a well-loved car that has taken some rough roads. Cardiac rehabilitation (or *"cardiac rehab"* for short) is like a top-notch mechanic shop for your heart, except you are not just fixing it—you are upgrading it. This program does not just help you get back on the road; it teaches you how to navigate your health better so you can drive smoother and longer. Cardiac rehab is the gold standard for recovering from heart conditions (76, 77). It is a medically supervised program that combines exercise, education, and emotional support to help you rebuild strength, regain confidence, and reclaim your life. Think of it as a heart health boot camp where the focus is on you, your journey, and your future.

What Happens in Cardiac Rehab?

Let us start with the nuts and bolts. Cardiac rehab typically involves a multidisciplinary team of healthcare professionals—think doctors, nurses, physical therapists, and sometimes even dietitians and psychologists. This dream team crafts a personalized plan just for you. Your program starts with a thorough assessment. They will check your heart health, fitness level, and any other medical concerns. Based on this, they will design an exercise routine that is safe, effective, and tailored to your needs.

Light Exercise with Big Benefits

The exercise component usually kicks off gently. Picture yourself walking on a treadmill or pedalling a stationary bike while a nurse keeps an eye on your heart rate and blood pressure. No one is going to ask you to run a marathon—this is about easing in and building up. As you progress, the intensity and duration of your workouts gradually increase, giving your heart a workout that is challenging but not overwhelming.

Strength Meets Stamina

In addition to cardio, you might engage in light resistance training. This helps strengthen your muscles, improve balance, and make daily activities easier. It is like giving your body the tools it needs to handle life with more ease and less strain on your heart.

Beyond the Treadmill

If you think cardiac rehab is just about breaking a sweat, think again. The education component is where the real magic happens.

Mastering Heart-Healthy Habits

You will learn the ABCs of heart health, from understanding your medications to recognizing signs of trouble. And let us talk food—your rehab team will teach you how to whip up meals that are not only delicious but also good for your ticker. Spoiler: you do not have to give up all your favourites, just tweak them a bit.

Stress Management 101

Stress is not just an emotional nuisance; it is a heavyweight when it comes to heart health. Cardiac rehab often includes techniques like mindfulness, meditation, or simple breathing exercises to help you manage stress effectively. Think of it as a mental spa day that your heart will love.

Lifestyle Changes That Stick

The key to a successful rehab journey is not just what you do during the program—it is about what you take with you afterward. You will learn practical tips to make exercise, healthy eating, and stress management a part of your everyday routine.

The Emotional Lift

Here is a little secret: cardiac rehab is not just for your heart—it is also for your soul. Recovering from a heart condition can feel isolating, but in cardiac rehab, you are not alone. You will meet others who are walking the same path, sharing similar challenges and triumphs. These connections can be a game-changer. Imagine swapping stories, cheering each other on, and finding comfort in knowing you are in this together. And let us not underestimate the power of encouragement from your healthcare team. Their guidance and positive reinforcement can boost your confidence and make you feel like a superhero.

Your Next Chapter

Graduating from cardiac rehab is not the finish line—it is the starting line of a new, healthier chapter in your life.

Staying Active

Keep the momentum going by incorporating regular exercise into your routine. Whether it is a morning walk, a yoga class, or dancing around your kitchen, find activities you enjoy and stick with them.

Healthy Eating Made Easy

Apply what you have learned about nutrition to create heart-healthy meals that you actually look forward to eating. Remember, it is not about perfection—it is about progress.

A Lifelong Commitment

The habits you build during cardiac rehab are tools for life. Keep using them to stay strong, prevent further heart issues, and enjoy the vibrant life you deserve.

Let Us Get Moving!

Exercise is medicine, and cardiac rehab is the prescription that keeps on giving. It is not just about strengthening your heart—it is about strengthening your confidence, independence, and zest for life. So, lace up those sneakers, grab a bottle of water, and take the first step. Whether it is a gentle walk or a heart-pumping bike ride, every move you make is a victory for your health. Remember, your heart is not just a muscle; it is the rhythm of your life. Treat it well, and it will beat stronger, longer, and happier—for you and the people you love.

CHAPTER 12: MEDICATIONS, FRAILTY, AND HEART DISEASE

Medications can be a double-edged sword. On one side, they save lives and manage symptoms. On the other, they can complicate things, especially when you are dealing with frailty and heart disease (94, 95). In this chapter, we will explore the tricky relationship between medications, frailty, and heart health, and how to navigate it without pulling your hair out.

12.1 Polypharmacy: Managing Multiple Medications

If you have ever felt like your pillbox looks more like a pharmacy shelf, you are not alone. Taking multiple medications—what doctors call "polypharmacy"—is common, especially as we age (96). While these meds often help, juggling too many can turn into a circus act. Let us dive into how to manage this medication juggling act effectively, keeping the balance between necessity and overload.

The Changing Body: Processing Medications as We Age

Here is the thing: as you get older, your body becomes less efficient at processing medications (97). Your liver slows down, your kidneys take a little longer to flush things out, and your frailty can make you more sensitive to side effects. Add heart disease to the mix, and it is easy for things to spiral out of control.

Imagine your body as a well-oiled machine that has been running smoothly for years. Over time, parts may wear out and need a bit more care to function properly. This is especially true for organs like the liver and kidneys, which play a crucial role in metabolizing and excreting medications. When these organs slow down, medications can linger in your system longer than intended, leading to potential side effects and interactions.

The Medication Balancing Act: Examples from Everyday Life

Take, for instance, blood pressure pills. They are great at keeping your heart safe but can sometimes cause dizziness or weakness, which might worsen frailty. Or diuretics, which help with fluid retention but can deplete potassium—a key mineral for muscle strength. It is a balancing act that requires careful monitoring and adjustment.

Imagine walking a tightrope while juggling flaming torches. That is what managing multiple medications can feel like. Each medication has its benefits and potential downsides, and the key is to balance them in a way that maximizes their positive effects while minimizing the negatives (98).

Tips for Managing Polypharmacy

So, how do you manage this medication juggling act? Here are some practical tips:

Know Your Meds: Keep a list of all the medications you take, including over-the-counter ones and supplements. This list should include the name of the medication, the dosage, and the reason you are taking it. Update this list regularly and share it with every healthcare provider you visit. Think of it as your medication passport—essential for safe travel through your healthcare journey.

Ask Questions: Do not be shy! If a medication has side effects that bother you, speak up. Ask your doctor or pharmacist about what to expect from your medications, how they should be taken, and what potential interactions might occur. Remember, there are no silly questions when it comes to your health. If a medication causes side effects that affect your quality of life, let your healthcare provider know. They might be able to adjust the dosage or suggest an alternative.

Simplify When Possible: Your doctor might be able to combine medications or adjust dosages to lighten the load. Sometimes, less is more. For instance, some medications come in combination forms, where a single pill contains two or more active ingredients. This can reduce the number of pills you need to take each day. Discuss with your doctor the possibility of simplifying your medication regimen.

Beware of Interactions: Some medications do not play well together. Make sure your healthcare provider knows about everything you are taking. This includes over-the-counter medications, herbal supplements, and vitamins. Certain combinations can cause harmful interactions, reducing the effectiveness of your medications or increasing the risk of side effects. Always double-check with your healthcare provider or pharmacist before adding a new medication to your routine.

Practical Strategies for Medication Management

Managing multiple medications can feel overwhelming, but there are practical strategies to make it easier:

Use a Pill Organizer: A pill organizer can help you keep track of your medications and ensure you are taking them at the right times. Choose one with compartments for different times of the day and fill it up at the beginning of each week.

Set Reminders: Use alarms or smartphone apps to remind you when it is time to take your medications. Consistency is key to managing your medications effectively.

Regular Check-Ins: Schedule regular check-ins with your healthcare provider to review your medications. These appointments are an opportunity to discuss any side effects, make adjustments, and ensure your medications are still the best choices for your health needs.

Stay Informed: Keep up-to-date with information about your medications. Read the information leaflets provided with your prescriptions, and do not hesitate to reach out to your healthcare provider with any questions or concerns.

Communicate: If you are seeing multiple healthcare providers, ensure they are all aware of your medication regimen. Coordination between your doctors can help prevent conflicts and ensure a cohesive approach to your treatment.

Empowering Yourself in Your Healthcare Journey

Remember, you are the boss of your healthcare team. If something feels off, it is okay to wave a red flag. Advocating for yourself is an important part of managing your health. By staying informed, asking questions, and working closely with your healthcare providers, you can navigate the complexities of polypharmacy with confidence.

Managing multiple medications does not have to be a circus act. With the right strategies and a proactive approach, you can keep everything in balance, ensuring your medications work effectively and safely. Here is to stay informed, empowered, and in control of your health!

12.2 How Frailty Alters Medication Effects

Ever notice how some people seem to handle strong medications like champions while others feel knocked out by a simple aspirin? Frailty is one reason why. When you are frail, your body's reserves—energy, strength, and resilience—are already running on low. Medications that might not bother a robust person can pack a bigger punch. Let us dive into why this happens and what you can do about it.

The Body's Reserve Tank: Running on Low

When you are frail, it is like your body is running on its reserve tank. Your energy levels, strength, and overall resilience are already compromised. Imagine trying to run a marathon with just a sip of water and a cracker—you are bound to hit a wall sooner than someone fully fuelled. This makes frail individuals more sensitive to medications, which can result in stronger side effects.

Blood Thinners: Double-Edged Swords

Take blood thinners, for example. These medications are life-saving for preventing strokes, but they can cause bleeding risks that frail individuals might not recover from as easily. For a robust person, a minor cut might just need a bandage. For someone who's frail, that same cut could lead to significant blood loss and complications.

Pain Medications: Tricky Territory

Pain medications, especially opioids, are another tricky area. Opioids, often prescribed for chronic pain, can cause dizziness, confusion, and even falls—a dangerous combo for anyone, let alone someone dealing with frailty and heart disease. Imagine feeling like you are perpetually on a merry-go-round, dizzy and unsteady. This can lead to falls, which are particularly dangerous for frail individuals due to their lower bone density and slower healing rates.

The Metabolism Maze

And it is not just about the medications themselves; it is about how your body processes them. Frailty can slow metabolism and change how drugs are absorbed, distributed, and eliminated. This means even a "normal" dose might feel too strong. It is like your body's usual conveyor belt system is on the fritz, processing everything at a snail's pace, which can lead to an accumulation of the drug in your system.

What Can You Do?

Managing medication effects when you are frail requires a proactive and informed approach. Here are some strategies to help you navigate this complex landscape:

Start Low, Go Slow: When starting a new medication, doctors often recommend beginning with the lowest possible dose and increasing gradually. This approach minimizes the risk of overwhelming your system and helps identify the right dosage without causing adverse effects. Think of it as dipping your toes in the water before diving in.

Monitor Closely: Keep track of how you feel after starting a new medication. Note any side effects, changes in energy, appetite, or mood. Maintain a medication diary to document these observations and share them with your doctor. This helps your healthcare provider make informed adjustments to your treatment plan.

Be Honest: If a medication makes you feel lousy, speak up. Your doctor can adjust the dosage or switch to a different medication that might be better tolerated. Remember, you are the expert on how you feel, and your feedback is crucial in finding the best treatment for you.

Managing Common Side Effects

Different medications come with their own sets of side effects. Here is how you can manage some common ones:

Dizziness and Light-headedness: If you experience dizziness, try to stand up slowly, especially after lying down or sitting. Drinking plenty of fluids and avoiding sudden movements can also help. If dizziness persists, consult your doctor.

Digestive Issues: Some medications can cause nausea, vomiting, or constipation. Eating small, frequent meals and staying hydrated can mitigate these effects. For constipation, include high-fiber foods in your diet and consider a gentle stool softener if recommended by your doctor.

Fatigue: Feeling unusually tired? Ensure you are getting enough rest and pacing your activities throughout the day. Sometimes, adjusting the timing of your medication can help. Discuss any persistent fatigue with your healthcare provider.

Mood Changes: If you notice changes in your mood or experience anxiety, depression, or irritability, do not hesitate to talk to your doctor. They might adjust your medication or recommend additional support, such as counseling.

Practical Tips for Medication Management

Stay Organized: Use a pill organizer to keep track of your medications and ensure you are taking them correctly. A weekly organizer with compartments for each day can be a lifesaver.

Set Reminders: Use alarms or smartphone apps to remind you when it is time to take your medication. Consistency is key to maintaining the effectiveness of your treatment.

Regular Check-Ins: Schedule regular check-ins with your healthcare provider to review your medications and discuss any concerns. These appointments are an opportunity to make necessary adjustments and ensure your medications are working as intended.

Stay Informed: Educate yourself about your medications. Read the information leaflets provided with your prescriptions and do not hesitate to ask your doctor or pharmacist questions. Knowledge empowers you to make informed decisions about your treatment.

Empowering Yourself in Your Healthcare Journey

Medications are meant to improve your quality of life; not make you feel worse. Do not settle for less. By being proactive, informed, and communicative, you can manage your medications effectively and ensure they support your health goals. Remember, you are in the driver's seat when it comes to your healthcare. If something feels off, it is okay to wave a red flag and advocate for yourself. With the right strategies and support, you can navigate the complexities of medication management and maintain your health and well-being.

In summary, frailty affects how your body tolerates medications, but with careful management and open communication with your healthcare provider, you can find a balance that works for you. Here is to taking charge of your health and ensuring that your medications enhance, rather than hinder, your quality of life!

12.3 Medication Strategies To Protect Heart Health

Let us talk about medications specifically designed to keep your heart healthy. From blood pressure pills to cholesterol-lowering statins, these drugs are vital—but they need a little extra TLC when frailty enters the picture. Let us dive deeper into how these medications work, their potential side effects, and practical strategies to manage them effectively.

Blood Pressure Medications: Balancing Act

High blood pressure is a big risk factor for heart disease, but aggressive treatment can sometimes go too far, especially in frail individuals. Low blood pressure might make you feel lightheaded, increasing the risk of falls. The goal is not perfection—it is balance.

Types of Blood Pressure Medications

Angiotensin-Converting Enzyme (ACE) Inhibitors: These relax blood vessels and reduce the workload on the heart. Common side effects include a dry cough and increased potassium levels.

Angiotensin II Receptor Blockers (ARBs): ARBs, are a vital class of medications for heart health, particularly for individuals with frailty. They work similarly to ACE inhibitors by relaxing blood vessels and lowering blood pressure but without some of the common side effects like a persistent cough.

Diuretics: These help the body eliminate excess salt and water. They are great for reducing blood pressure but can lead to dehydration and low potassium levels. Diuretics are used to manage fluid retention in conditions like heart failure and can be lifesavers. However, they can also deplete potassium and other electrolytes, leading to muscle weakness. Eating potassium-rich foods (hello, bananas, and spinach!) can help. Common diuretics:

Furosemide: A potent diuretic that can quickly reduce fluid buildup but may lead to dehydration.

Hydrochlorothiazide: Often used for hypertension and less intense fluid reduction, but still requires monitoring of electrolyte levels.

Think of diuretics as your body's natural drain, helping to get rid of excess water. Just be sure to replenish those essential electrolytes by eating foods rich in potassium like bananas, oranges, spinach, and potatoes. And do not forget to stay hydrated!

Calcium channel blockers: Calcium channel blockers are another key class of medications used to protect heart health, especially in individuals with frailty. They work by relaxing the blood vessels and reducing the heart's workload, making it easier for the heart to pump blood. However, like all medications, calcium channel blockers come with their own set of potential side effects. These can include: swelling in the ankles and feet, dizziness or light-headedness, constipation, and headaches. For frail individuals, these side effects can be more pronounced, so it is important to monitor how you feel after starting or adjusting a calcium channel blocker.

Beta-Blockers: These reduce heart rate and blood pressure. Side effects can include fatigue and dizziness.

Imagine trying to walk a tightrope—balance is key. You need to keep your blood pressure in check without tipping over into low blood pressure territory. This is where your healthcare provider comes in, adjusting dosages and medications to find the sweet spot.

Cholesterol Medications: Rock Stars of Prevention

Statins are the rock stars of heart disease prevention. They lower bad cholesterol and reduce inflammation. But for frail individuals, side effects like muscle pain can be problematic. If you are on a statin and feel achy, do not suffer in silence—there are alternatives. Common statins are:

Atorvastatin: Known for its potency in lowering LDL cholesterol. Muscle pain is a common side effect.

Simvastatin: Effective but may interact with other medications, increasing the risk of side effects.

Rosuvastatin: Often recommended for its efficacy and relatively lower risk of muscle pain.

Think of statins as your body's internal cleanup crew, sweeping away bad cholesterol. However, if the crew starts causing too much commotion (muscle pain), it is time to talk to your doctor about other options, which can lower cholesterol without the same risk of muscle pain.

Blood Thinners: Double-Edged Swords

Blood thinners are crucial for preventing strokes and managing heart rhythm issues like atrial fibrillation. But they also carry bleeding risks. For frail adults, regular check-ins with your doctor are essential to strike the right balance. Types of blood thinners are:

Warfarin (Coumadin): Requires regular blood tests to monitor levels and adjust dosage. Dietary restrictions (like avoiding too much vitamin K) apply.

Direct Oral Anticoagulants (DOACs): Include medications like apixaban and rivaroxaban. They do not require regular blood tests but can still pose bleeding risks. Imagine blood thinners as a double-edged sword—they can prevent clots but also make you more prone to bleeding. It is crucial to follow your doctor's instructions and report any unusual bruising or bleeding immediately.

Practical Medication Tips for Heart Health

Managing heart medications can feel overwhelming, but a few strategies can make it easier:

Take Them at the Same Time Daily: Build a routine around meals or bedtime. Consistency helps maintain stable levels of medication in your body, improving efficacy and reducing the risk of missed doses.

Invest in a Pill Organizer: It is a game-changer for keeping track of multiple meds. Choose one with compartments for different times of the day to avoid confusion and ensure you are taking the right doses at the right times.

Schedule Regular Reviews: Medications should evolve as your health changes. Your doctor can help adjust doses or stop ones that are no longer needed. Think of it as spring cleaning for your medication list—out with the old, in with the new!

Stay Educated: Understand why you are taking each medication. Knowledge is power! Read the information leaflets, ask your doctor questions, and stay informed about how each medication supports your health. The more you know, the better you can manage your treatment.

Communicate: Do not hesitate to communicate with your healthcare team about any concerns or side effects. Open communication ensures that your treatment plan remains effective and safe.

Be Mindful of Interactions: Some medications can interact with each other, affecting how they work. Always inform your healthcare provider about all the medications you are taking, including over-the-counter drugs and supplements.

Proper medication management is a powerful tool in the fight against frailty and heart disease. With a thoughtful approach, they can help you live a longer, healthier life. Take charge, stay informed, and remember: your health is a partnership between you and your healthcare team. In the words of a wise pharmacist: "Pills don't work unless you take them." But just as important? Taking the right ones in the right way. You have got this!

CHAPTER 13: MENTAL HEALTH, FRAILTY, AND HEART DISEASE

Mental health plays a crucial role in the lives of those with frailty and heart disease (99). It is not just about keeping your body in tip-top shape; your mind needs some love too. In this chapter, we will explore the intricate connections between frailty, depression, stress, and cardiovascular risk. Plus, we will dive into holistic approaches that can boost mental well-being. Let us get to the heart of the matter!

13.1 The Frailty-Depression Link

Depression and frailty often go hand in hand, creating a vicious cycle that can be tough to break (100, 101). When you are frail, your body's reserves are low, and even the simplest tasks can feel overwhelming. This constant struggle can lead to feelings of sadness, hopelessness, and fatigue—classic symptoms of depression. But the relationship goes both ways: depression can also make you more vulnerable to frailty.

The Body-Mind Connection

Imagine depression as a fog that clouds your mind, making everything seem harder and less enjoyable. When you are already dealing with the physical limitations of frailty, this mental fog can intensify your feelings of helplessness. Depression can sap your motivation to stay active, eat well, and take care of yourself—all of which are crucial for managing frailty and heart disease.

Think of it this way: your body and mind are like dance partners. If one stumbles, the other is likely to follow. Depression can make your body feel heavier and harder to move, while frailty can make your mind feel sluggish and uninspired.

Common Symptoms

Depression in frail individuals might not always look the same as it does in younger or healthier people. Keep an eye out for these signs:

Persistent Sadness or Anxiety: Feeling down or excessively worried without clear reasons.

Loss of Interest in Activities: Things that used to bring joy no longer seem enjoyable.

Changes in Appetite or Weight: Either eating too much or too little, leading to weight changes.

Trouble Sleeping or Sleeping Too Much: Insomnia or excessive sleeping can both be signs of depression.

Fatigue or Low Energy: Feeling tired all the time, even with enough rest.

Difficulty Concentrating or Making Decisions: Trouble focusing on tasks or making everyday choices.

These symptoms can be subtle but have a profound impact on your daily life. It is essential to pay attention to these changes and take them seriously.

Breaking the Cycle

Breaking the cycle of frailty and depression is challenging, but it is possible with the right approach. Here are some strategies to help you tackle both issues simultaneously:

Medication: Antidepressants can help balance the chemicals in your brain that affect mood. Your doctor can help determine the right medication and dosage for you. It might take some time to find the perfect fit, but it is worth the effort.

Psychological treatments: Psychological treatments for depression are designed to help individuals manage and overcome their symptoms through various therapeutic approaches. Each person's experience with depression is unique, so it is important to work with a mental health professional to find the treatment that works best for you. Combining psychological treatments with lifestyle changes, social support, and, if necessary, medication, can lead to a comprehensive and effective approach to managing depression.

Lifestyle Changes: Incorporating small, manageable changes into your daily routine can have a significant impact on both your physical and mental health:

Physical Activity: Even gentle exercises like walking, stretching, or yoga can boost your mood and help you regain strength. Aim for at least 30 minutes of activity most days of the week. Physical activity releases endorphins, which are natural mood lifters.

Balanced Diet: Eating a nutritious diet can support brain health and improve your overall well-being. Include plenty of fruits, vegetables, whole grains, lean proteins, and healthy fats in your meals. Omega-3 fatty acids, found in fish and flaxseeds, are particularly beneficial for mental health.

Sleep Hygiene: Establishing a regular sleep routine can improve the quality of your rest and help regulate your mood. Create a calming bedtime environment, avoid caffeine and electronics before bed, and try to go to sleep and wake up at the same time each day.

Social Connections: Building and maintaining strong social connections is vital for mental health, especially for individuals dealing with frailty and heart disease. Think of social connections as the glue that holds the pieces of your life together, providing emotional support, reducing feelings of isolation, and enhancing overall well-being. Why social connections matter (102, 103) is an important question. Humans are inherently social creatures. We thrive on interaction, support, and a sense of belonging.

For frail individuals, social connections can offer the following benefits:

Emotional Support: Sharing your experiences, fears, and joys with others can provide a sense of relief and comfort. Emotional support from friends and family can help you navigate the challenges of frailty and heart disease.

Reduced Isolation: Isolation can intensify feelings of depression and anxiety. Staying connected with others can combat loneliness and promote a more positive outlook on life.

Improved Mental Health: Regular social interactions can boost your mood, reduce stress, and improve cognitive function. Engaging with others keeps your mind active and engaged.

Encouragement and Motivation: Friends and family can encourage you to stay active, eat well, and adhere to your medication regimen. They can also provide a sense of accountability, motivating you to take better care of yourself.

Ways to Foster Social Connections

Here are some practical ways to build and maintain strong social connections:

Join Support Groups: Connecting with others who are going through similar experiences can be incredibly comforting and encouraging. Support groups offer a sense of community and understanding. Look for local or online groups focused on frailty, heart disease, or general senior support.

Spend Time with Loved Ones: Regularly spending time with friends and family can boost your mood and provide a sense of belonging. Plan regular get-togethers, whether it is a weekly dinner, a phone call, or a virtual meetup. These interactions can help you feel more connected and supported.

Volunteer: Volunteering can provide a sense of purpose and fulfillment. It is also a great way to meet new people and make a positive impact in your community. Look for volunteer opportunities that match your interests and abilities.

Engage in Hobbies: Finding meaningful activities can give you a sense of purpose and satisfaction. Join clubs or groups that share your interests, whether it is gardening, knitting, book clubs, or walking groups. These activities provide an opportunity to connect with others who share your passions.

Use Technology: If in-person interactions are difficult, consider using technology to stay connected. Video calls, social media, and online forums can help you maintain relationships and build new ones. Virtual meetups can be just as meaningful and provide a sense of connection.

Overcoming Barriers to Social Connection

For frail individuals, there may be barriers to social connection, such as limited mobility, health issues, or anxiety. Here are some strategies to overcome these challenges:

Transportation Assistance: If mobility is an issue, look for community services that offer transportation assistance for seniors. Friends or family members may also be willing to help with rides to social events or appointments.

Accessible Activities: Choose activities that are accessible and suitable for your physical abilities. Many community centers offer programs specifically designed for seniors or those with limited mobility.

Online Communities: If leaving the house is challenging, explore online communities and virtual events. These can provide a sense of connection without the need for physical travel.

Communicate Your Needs: Let your friends and family know if you need assistance or accommodations to participate in social activities. They may be able to help in ways you had not considered.

The Importance of Balance

While social connections are important, it is also crucial to find a balance that works for you. It is okay to take time for yourself and rest when needed. Listen to your body and mind, and do not hesitate to set boundaries if you feel overwhelmed.

Taking the First Step

Taking the first step to address both frailty and depression can feel daunting, but it is crucial for your overall health and well-being. Remember, you do not have to do it alone. Reach out to your healthcare provider, mental health professional, or a trusted loved one for support. By addressing both physical and mental health, you can break the cycle of frailty and depression and improve your quality of life. It is about finding a balance that works for you and making small, sustainable changes that support your overall well-being.

Start small, whether it is reaching out to a friend for a chat, joining an online group, or participating in a local event. Every little effort counts and can make a significant difference in your mental and emotional well-being. Remember, you do not have to do it all at once. Focus on one or two strategies that resonate with you and gradually expand your social network. Over time, you will find that these connections enrich your life and provide the support you need to thrive.

In summary, social connections are a vital component of mental health, especially for individuals dealing with frailty and heart disease. By fostering strong relationships and staying engaged with others, you can enhance your quality of life and build a robust support system. Here is to connect, supporting, and thriving together!

13.2 Stress And Cardiovascular Risk

Stress is like adding gasoline to a fire when it comes to heart disease. Chronic stress can lead to a host of problems that put your heart at risk, including high blood pressure, inflammation, and unhealthy behaviors like smoking or overeating. For frail individuals, the impact of stress can be even more pronounced. Let us dive into the practical details of how stress affects the heart and what you can do about it.

The Stress-Heart Disease Connection

Stress triggers the release of hormones like cortisol and adrenaline, which prepare your body for a "fight or flight" response. While this response is helpful in short bursts—like if you are running late for an appointment—chronic stress keeps your body in a constant state of alert. This prolonged state of readiness can lead to high blood pressure, increased heart rate, and inflammation—all of which are bad news for your heart (22, 104).

Imagine your body as a car engine revving constantly. Over time, this continuous strain wears down the engine's parts, leading to damage. Similarly, chronic stress keeps your heart working overtime, which can lead to wear and tear on your cardiovascular system.

Symptoms of Chronic Stress

Recognizing the symptoms of chronic stress is the first step to managing it. Symptoms can include:

Headaches: Tension headaches are common, often manifesting as a dull, persistent ache around the forehead or the back of the head and neck.

Muscle Tension or Pain: Chronic stress can cause muscles to tense up, leading to pain and discomfort, particularly in the shoulders, neck, and back.

Chest Pain or Rapid Heartbeat: Stress can cause palpitations or a feeling of tightness in the chest, which can be alarming and mimic heart attack symptoms.

Fatigue: Persistent stress can drain your energy, making you feel constantly tired and worn out.

Trouble Sleeping: Stress can interfere with your sleep, causing insomnia or unrestful sleep, which further exacerbates fatigue.

Irritability or Mood Swings: Chronic stress can impact your emotional state, leading to irritability, anxiety, or sudden mood swings.

These symptoms can significantly impact your quality of life and increase your risk of heart disease. Recognizing and addressing these symptoms early is crucial for maintaining your heart health.

Managing Stress

Managing stress effectively can lower your cardiovascular risk and improve your overall well-being. Here are some strategies to consider:

Exercise: Physical activity can reduce stress hormones and release endorphins, the body's natural mood lifters. Even a short daily walk can make a difference. Think of exercise as your body's natural stress buster. Whether it is a gentle walk, a yoga session, or a dance class, moving your body can help clear your mind and improve your mood.

Relaxation Techniques: Practices like deep breathing, meditation, tai chi, and yoga can calm your mind and reduce stress. These techniques help you focus on the present moment and let go of worries. Imagine taking a mental vacation every day—these practices can help you find peace amidst the chaos. You can also practice mindfulness. Mindfulness practices involve paying attention to the present moment without judgment. Meditation, in particular, can help calm the mind and reduce stress. Set aside a few minutes each day to practice mindfulness or meditation. There are many guided meditation apps available that can help you get started.

Social Support: Spending time with loved ones, joining support groups, or talking to a therapist can provide emotional support and help you cope with stress. Social interactions can offer a sense of connection and belonging, reducing feelings of isolation and loneliness.

Healthy Habits: Eating a balanced diet, getting enough sleep, and avoiding unhealthy coping mechanisms like smoking or excessive drinking can also help manage stress. Your body needs proper fuel and rest to combat stress effectively. Aim for a diet rich in fruits, vegetables, whole grains, and lean proteins, and establish a regular sleep routine.

Time Management: Organizing your schedule and setting realistic goals can reduce the feeling of being overwhelmed. Prioritize tasks, break them into manageable steps, and take regular breaks. Remember, it is okay to say no to additional responsibilities if you are feeling stretched thin.

Hobbies and Interests: Engaging in activities you enjoy can provide a much-needed break from stress. Whether it is gardening, painting, reading, or playing a musical instrument, hobbies can bring joy and relaxation into your life.

Professional Support: Sometimes, managing stress on your own can be challenging. Seeking help from a mental health professional, such as a therapist or counsellor, can provide valuable support and coping strategies. Cognitive behavioral therapy (CBT) is particularly effective for managing stress and anxiety.

Making Stress Management a Habit

Incorporating stress management techniques into your daily routine can have a profound impact on your overall well-being. Here are some tips to make stress management a regular part of your life:

Start Small: Choose one or two stress management techniques that resonate with you and incorporate them into your daily routine. Gradually add more practices as you become comfortable with them.

Consistency is Key: Make stress management a priority by scheduling time for it each day. Consistency helps build healthy habits that can lead to lasting changes.

Listen to Your Body: Pay attention to how your body responds to stress and the techniques you are using. Adjust your practices as needed to find what works best for you.

Stay Flexible: Life is unpredictable, and stressors can change. Be open to trying new stress management techniques and adapting your routine to meet your current needs.

Seek Support: Do not hesitate to reach out for help if you are struggling with stress. Friends, family, and mental health professionals can provide valuable support and guidance.

By taking proactive steps to manage stress, you can lower your cardiovascular risk, improve your overall well-being, and enhance your quality of life. Remember, managing stress is an ongoing process, and small, consistent efforts can lead to significant improvements over time.

In summary, stress is a significant risk factor for heart disease, but with effective management strategies, you can reduce its impact on your heart and overall health. Incorporate these techniques into your daily routine and take control of your well-being. Your heart will thank you for it!

13.3 Holistic Approaches To Mental Well-Being

A holistic approach to mental well-being considers the whole person—body, mind, and spirit (105). For individuals with frailty and heart disease, this approach can provide comprehensive support that addresses both physical, mental, social and spiritual health (106). By focusing on mind-body practices, nutrition, sleep, social connections, and professional support, you can create a balanced and fulfilling lifestyle that promotes overall wellness.

Mind-Body Practices

Mind-body practices like mindfulness, meditation, and tai chi can help reduce stress, improve mood, and enhance overall well-being. These practices encourage you to focus on the present moment, letting go of worries about the past or future. Regular practice can lead to lasting changes in how you respond to stress and improve your quality of life.

Mindfulness: Mindfulness involves paying attention to the present moment without judgment. By practicing mindfulness, you can become more aware of your thoughts and feelings, helping you manage them more effectively. Imagine taking a mental snapshot of the present, appreciating the sights, sounds, and sensations around you.

Meditation: Meditation is a practice that encourages you to focus your mind and achieve a state of relaxation and clarity. There are many forms of meditation, such as guided meditation, mantra meditation, and loving-kindness meditation. Even just a few minutes a day can make a difference. Think of it as giving your mind a mini-vacation.

Tai Chi: Tai chi is a gentle form of exercise that combines slow, flowing movements with deep breathing and meditation. It is often described as "meditation in motion" and can improve balance, flexibility, and mental clarity. Picture yourself moving gracefully like a flowing river, letting go of stress with each movement.

Prayer and Spiritual Practices: Religiosity, involving prayer and rituals, is linked to better health and quality of life. Many people worldwide see spirituality as vital to healing, alongside modern medicine. While spirituality reflects personal beliefs about a higher power that shape life choices and health, religiosity provides structure to those beliefs. Religious practices not only support spiritual well-being but also improve physical health and longevity. Emerging research in Neurotheology explores how spirituality might influence the brain and body (107), though this topic goes beyond this book's focus.

Nutrition and Mental Health

What you eat can have a significant impact on your mental health. A balanced diet rich in fruits, vegetables, whole grains, and lean proteins can support brain function and improve mood (11). Omega-3 fatty acids, found in fish, like salmon, and in flaxseeds, are particularly beneficial for mental health.

Fruits and Vegetables: These nutrient-dense foods provide essential vitamins and minerals that support brain health. Aim to fill half your plate with a variety of colorful fruits and vegetables at each meal. Think of them as nature's multivitamins, packed with everything you need to keep your mind sharp.

Whole Grains: Whole grains like brown rice, quinoa, and oats provide steady energy and support cognitive function. They are the complex carbs that keep your brain fuelled throughout the day. Swap out refined grains for whole grains to maximize their benefits.

Lean Proteins: Protein is essential for the production of neurotransmitters, the chemicals that transmit signals in your brain. Include sources like chicken, fish, beans, and tofu in your diet. Imagine proteins as the building blocks for your brain's communication system.

Omega-3 Fatty Acids: These healthy fats are important for brain health and can help reduce symptoms of depression and anxiety. Include fatty fish, walnuts, chia seeds, and flaxseeds in your diet. Picture omega-3s as the lubricants that keep your brain's gears turning smoothly.

Sleep and Recovery

Good sleep is essential for mental well-being (108). When you are well-rested, you are better able to manage stress and handle life's challenges. Establish a regular sleep routine, create a calming bedtime environment, and avoid caffeine and electronic devices before bed to improve sleep quality.

Regular Sleep Routine: Go to bed and wake up at the same time each day, even on weekends. This helps regulate your body's internal clock and improves the quality of your sleep. Think of it as setting a consistent schedule for your brain's nightly rest and recovery.

Calming Bedtime Environment: Create a relaxing environment in your bedroom. Keep the room cool, dark, and quiet. Use comfortable bedding and eliminate any sources of light or noise that might disturb your sleep. Imagine your bedroom as a sanctuary dedicated to rest and relaxation.

Avoid Caffeine and Electronics: Caffeine and electronic devices can interfere with your ability to fall asleep. Avoid consuming caffeine in the afternoon and evening and limit your use of electronic devices before bed. Picture yourself winding down with a good book or a warm bath instead.

Social Connections

Humans are social creatures, and maintaining strong social connections is vital for mental health (109). Spending time with family and friends, joining clubs or community groups, and volunteering can help you feel connected and supported. If in-person interactions are difficult, consider virtual meetups or phone calls.

Spending Time with Loved Ones: Regularly connecting with family and friends can provide emotional support and reduce feelings of isolation. Plan regular get-togethers, phone calls, or video chats to stay connected. Think of these interactions as emotional nourishment for your soul.

Joining Clubs or Community Groups: Engaging in activities and hobbies with others can provide a sense of belonging and purpose. Look for local clubs or groups that align with your interests, whether it is gardening, knitting, or reading. Imagine these groups as your personal support network.

Volunteering: Giving back to your community can provide a sense of fulfillment and help you build new relationships. Find volunteer opportunities that match your skills and passions. Picture yourself making a positive impact while connecting with like-minded individuals.

Therapy and Counseling

Talking to a mental health professional can provide valuable support and guidance. Therapy can help you develop coping strategies, address underlying issues, and improve your overall mental health. Cognitive-behavioral therapy (CBT), in particular, is effective for treating depression and anxiety.

Cognitive-Behavioral Therapy (CBT): CBT focuses on identifying and changing negative thought patterns and behaviors. It is a practical, goal-oriented approach that can help you develop healthier ways of thinking and reacting. Think of it as a mental workout, strengthening your ability to handle life's challenges.

Supportive Counseling: Sometimes, simply talking to someone who listens and understands can make a world of difference. Supportive counseling provides a safe space to express your feelings and receive empathy and encouragement. Picture your therapist as a trusted guide on your journey to mental well-being.

Taking Charge of Your Mental Health

Taking a proactive approach to your mental health is essential, especially when dealing with frailty and heart disease. By recognizing the signs of depression and stress, seeking support, and adopting holistic practices, you can improve your mental well-being and enhance your overall quality of life.

Recognizing the Signs: Pay attention to changes in your mood, energy levels, and overall well-being. Early recognition of stress and depression can help you seek timely support and intervention.

Seeking Support: Do not hesitate to reach out to friends, family, or mental health professionals when you need help. Building a strong support network can provide emotional and practical assistance.

Adopting Holistic Practices: Incorporate mind-body practices, balanced nutrition, good sleep habits, and social connections into your daily routine. These holistic practices can create a foundation for lasting mental well-being.

Remember, your mind and body are interconnected (110). Taking care of your mental health can have a positive impact on your physical health, and vice versa. By adopting a holistic approach, you can create a balanced and fulfilling lifestyle that supports both your mental and physical well-being. Here is to a healthier, happier you!

In brief, holistic approaches to mental well-being consider the whole person and provide comprehensive support for both physical and mental health. By focusing on mind-body practices, nutrition, sleep, social connections, and professional support, you can enhance your overall quality of life and build a strong foundation for a healthier future. Let us embrace a holistic lifestyle and thrive together!

CHAPTER 14: FRAIL WOMEN AND HEART DISEASE

Frailty and heart disease can affect anyone, but women often experience these conditions differently than men (111, 112). Understanding these differences is essential for effective prevention and care. Let us explore why women experience frailty and heart disease differently, the role of hormonal changes, and tailored approaches to prevention and care.

14.1 Why Women Experience Frailty And Heart Disease Differently

Women and men may share the same planet, but when it comes to frailty and heart disease, they often inhabit different worlds. The biological, social, and behavioral differences between the sexes mean that women face unique challenges.

Biological Differences

Women's bodies are built differently. They generally have smaller hearts and narrower blood vessels, which can affect how heart disease develops and presents. For example, women are more likely to experience microvascular disease, where the small blood vessels in the heart are damaged, leading to chest pain and other symptoms without the typical blockages seen in men's larger arteries (113, 114).

Hormonal Influences

Hormones, particularly estrogen, play a significant role in women's heart health. Estrogen has protective effects on the cardiovascular system, helping to maintain the flexibility of blood vessels and reduce inflammation (115, 116). However, during menopause, estrogen levels drop. Menopause is a natural biological process that marks the end of a woman's menstrual cycles. It typically occurs between the ages of 45 and 55, signifying the end of the reproductive years. This transition is confirmed after 12 consecutive months without a menstrual period. During this time, the body undergoes hormonal changes, which can lead to various symptoms such as hot flashes, mood swings, and changes in sleep patterns. It is a normal part of aging and a new phase of life. This hormonal shift can lead to changes in blood pressure, cholesterol levels, and body fat distribution—all of which contribute to cardiovascular risk (115) as well as frailty.

Differences in Symptoms

Women often experience heart disease symptoms differently than men (117, 118). While men typically report the classic symptom of chest pain, women may experience subtler signs such as shortness of breath, nausea, fatigue, and back or jaw pain. These atypical symptoms can lead to delays in diagnosis and treatment.

Social and Behavioral Factors

Social and behavioral factors also play a role. Women are more likely to be caregivers, juggling multiple roles and responsibilities, which can lead to chronic stress. This stress can exacerbate frailty and increase the risk of heart disease (13, 119). Additionally, women are more likely to experience depression and anxiety, which are linked to both frailty and heart disease.

Access to Healthcare

There are also differences in how women access and receive healthcare. Historically, medical research and treatment guidelines have been based primarily on men, leading to gaps in knowledge about women's health. Women may also be less likely to seek medical help for heart-related symptoms, either due to societal norms or because they prioritize their family's health over their own (120, 121).

Understanding the Impact

Understanding these differences is crucial for developing effective prevention and treatment strategies for women. Recognizing the unique symptoms, risk factors, and challenges women face can lead to better outcomes and improved quality of life.

14.2 Hormonal Changes And Heart Health

Hormonal changes, particularly those related to menopause, have a profound impact on women's heart health. Let us delve into how these hormonal shifts affect the cardiovascular system and what women can do to protect their hearts during these changes.

The Role of Estrogen

Estrogen is a hormone that plays a protective role in women's heart health (115). It helps maintain the flexibility and elasticity of blood vessels, reduces inflammation, and supports healthy cholesterol levels. Estrogen's beneficial effects help lower the risk of developing atherosclerosis (the buildup of plaque in the arteries) and other cardiovascular conditions .

Menopause and Heart Health

During menopause, which typically occurs between the ages of 45 and 55, women's estrogen levels decline significantly. This reduction in estrogen can have several adverse effects on heart health (116):

Increased Blood Pressure: Estrogen helps keep blood vessels relaxed. When levels drop, blood vessels can become stiffer and less flexible, leading to increased blood pressure.

Changes in Cholesterol Levels: Estrogen helps maintain healthy cholesterol levels. Postmenopause, women often experience higher levels of LDL (bad) cholesterol and lower levels of HDL (good) cholesterol, increasing the risk of heart disease.

Weight Gain and Fat Distribution: Hormonal changes during menopause can lead to weight gain and changes in fat distribution, particularly increased abdominal fat. This central obesity is a significant risk factor for heart disease.

Insulin Sensitivity: Declining estrogen levels can affect insulin sensitivity, leading to an increased risk of developing type 2 diabetes mellitus, which is a major risk factor for heart disease.

Managing Hormonal Changes

Managing the impact of hormonal changes during menopause on heart health involves a combination of lifestyle modifications and medical interventions (122):

Healthy Diet: Eating a balanced diet rich in fruits, vegetables, whole grains, lean proteins, and healthy fats can support heart health and mitigate the effects of hormonal changes. Foods high in phytoestrogens, such as soy products, flaxseeds, and legumes, may help mimic the effects of estrogen in the body.

Regular Exercise: Physical activity helps maintain a healthy weight, reduce blood pressure, and improve cholesterol levels. Aim for at least 150 minutes of moderate-intensity exercise per week, such as brisk walking, swimming, or cycling.

Stress Management: Chronic stress can exacerbate the effects of hormonal changes. Practices like mindfulness, meditation, yoga, and deep breathing exercises can help manage stress and improve overall well-being.

Medical Interventions: In some cases, hormone replacement therapy (HRT) may be recommended to alleviate menopausal symptoms and protect heart health. It is essential to discuss the risks and benefits of HRT with a healthcare provider to determine if it is the right option for you.

Regular Check-Ups: Regular medical check-ups are crucial for monitoring heart health and managing risk factors. Blood pressure, cholesterol levels, and blood sugar should be regularly assessed, and any changes should be addressed promptly.

14.3 Tailored Approaches To Prevention And Care

Given the unique ways in which women experience frailty and heart disease, tailored approaches to prevention and care are essential. Let us explore strategies that can help women maintain heart health and reduce frailty.

Personalized Risk Assessment

Individualized risk assessments can help identify specific factors that contribute to frailty and heart disease in women. These assessments should consider family history, hormonal status, lifestyle factors, and existing health conditions. By understanding each woman's unique risk profile, healthcare providers can develop personalized prevention and treatment plans.

Lifestyle Modifications

Lifestyle modifications play a crucial role in preventing frailty and heart disease. Here are some strategies that can make a significant difference:

Healthy Eating: Focus on a heart-healthy diet that includes plenty of fruits, vegetables, whole grains, lean proteins, and healthy fats. Limit the intake of processed foods, sugary beverages, and high-sodium snacks. Incorporate foods rich in antioxidants and anti-inflammatory properties, such as berries, nuts, and green leafy vegetables.

Physical Activity: Regular exercise is essential for maintaining cardiovascular health and reducing frailty. Aim for a mix of aerobic exercises, strength training, and flexibility exercises. Activities like walking, dancing, swimming, and yoga can be enjoyable and effective ways to stay active.

Stress Management: Managing stress is critical for heart health. Incorporate stress-reducing practices like mindfulness, meditation, deep breathing exercises, and hobbies that bring joy and relaxation. Establishing a routine that includes time for self-care can help manage stress levels effectively.

Sleep Hygiene: Prioritize good sleep hygiene by maintaining a regular sleep schedule, creating a calming bedtime routine, and ensuring a comfortable sleep environment. Quality sleep is essential for overall health and well-being.

Avoiding Harmful Behaviors: Avoid smoking and limit alcohol consumption, as these behaviors can significantly increase the risk of heart disease and other health issues.

Healthcare and Support

Access to healthcare and support is vital for women in managing frailty and heart disease. Here are some key considerations:

Regular Check-Ups: Regular medical check-ups allow for early detection and management of risk factors. Blood pressure, cholesterol levels, blood sugar, and weight should be monitored regularly.

Screening and Diagnostics: Ensure that screenings and diagnostic tests are tailored to women's specific needs. This includes mammograms, bone density tests, Pap test for cervical cancer screening and heart disease screenings that consider the unique presentation of symptoms in women.

Patient Education: Educating women about the symptoms, risk factors, and prevention strategies for heart disease.

CHAPTER 15: PREVENTING FRAILTY TO PROTECT YOUR HEART

Frailty and heart disease go hand in hand more often than we would like, but the good news is that you are not powerless. With a bit of effort and a sprinkle of fun, you can plant seeds of resilience today that will bloom into a healthier tomorrow.

15.1 Building Resilience Through Lifestyle Choices

Let us start with the basics: resilience. It is not some magical trait you are either born with or not; it is like a muscle you can strengthen over time. And the beauty of it is that your body and heart play just as big a role in resilience as your mindset.

Food: The Fuel for Resilience

Think of your heart as the engine that powers your body. A luxury car would not run on cheap fuel, and neither should your heart. But before you sigh at the thought of tasteless health food, let us banish that myth. Healthy eating does not mean endless bowls of plain lettuce or dry chicken. Instead, imagine meals bursting with color and flavor—vibrant stir-fries, roasted vegetables drizzled with olive oil, or a juicy salmon fillet seasoned to perfection. Love dessert? Swap out the sugar-laden treats for fresh berries with a dollop of Greek yogurt and a drizzle of honey. Delicious and heart-smart!

Let us not forget hydration. Water is your body's unsung hero. Dehydration can leave you feeling sluggish, and guess what? That sluggishness can make it harder for your heart to do its job. Keep a water bottle handy and make sipping a habit.

Move It or Lose It

When it comes to resilience, staying active is non-negotiable—but do not panic. You do not need to join a boot camp or train for the Olympics. Movement can be fun, and it does not have to be formal.

Have a dog? Take them for a brisk walk—it is good for both of you. Love music? Turn up the volume and dance like nobody's watching. Got a green thumb? Gardening counts as exercise, and bonus—it comes with built-in stress relief. If you want to take it up a notch, strength training is your best friend. No, I am not talking about bench-pressing 200 pounds at the gym. Even light weights or resistance bands can work wonders for your muscles and bones. Try lifting soup cans or doing squats while holding onto a chair for support. The key is consistency, not perfection. And do not forget balance exercises. Think of these as your secret weapon against frailty and falls. Practice standing on one leg while waiting for your coffee to brew or do simple stretches before bed.

Sleep: The Ultimate Recharge

Let us talk about sleep—the ultimate free health hack. Think of it as your body's nightly maintenance team, fixing the day's wear and tear while you snooze. If you are skimping on sleep, you are short-changing your heart and your resilience. Create a bedtime routine that feels luxurious. Dim the lights, read a calming book, or listen to soothing music. Skip the screens—yes, even your phone—for at least an hour before bed. And make your bedroom a haven: comfortable pillows, cool temperatures, and blackout curtains can work wonders. If you struggle to fall asleep, try this: take slow, deep breaths and focus on relaxing each part of your body, starting from your toes, and working upward. It is like sending a "chill out" message to your brain.

Friends: The Heart's Emotional Medicine

Here is a surprising resilience booster: your social life. Loneliness is not just a bummer; it is bad for your heart. Studies show that people with strong social ties tend to live longer and healthier lives (123, 124). So, how do you nurture your social circle? Start small. Invite a neighbour for a walk, join a community group, or catch up with an old friend over coffee. Do not have a group yet? Consider taking a class, volunteering, or even joining an online book club. And remember, laughter is great for your heart. Watch a funny movie, share a joke with a friend, or just let yourself giggle at life's little absurdities.

Stress: Taming the Silent Saboteur

Stress is sneaky—it can creep into your life and quietly wreak havoc on your heart and body. But with a few smart strategies, you can keep it in check.

Deep breathing is a game-changer. Whenever you feel tension rising, pause and take a few slow, deep breaths. Think of it as hitting the "reset" button for your mind and body. Another stress-buster? Gratitude. It might sound cheesy but writing down three things you are grateful for each day can shift your focus from what is wrong to what's right. It is like giving your brain a pep talk. And do not underestimate the power of mindfulness. Whether it is meditation, yoga, or simply savouring your morning coffee without distractions, being present in the moment can help you stay grounded.

The Bigger Picture

Building resilience through lifestyle choices is not about perfection—it is about progress. Start small, pick one or two habits to work on, and build from there. Each choice you make—whether it is swapping chips for nuts or walking instead of driving—adds up over time. So, take a deep breath, lace up your shoes, and grab a friend for a stroll. With every step, every bite, and every laugh, you are building a stronger, healthier you—and giving your heart the care it deserves.

15.2 How To Stay Active And Independent

Staying active does not mean you need to train for an Ironman competition or master the art of parkour. It is not about extremes—it is about doing what keeps you moving, feeling good, and enjoying life on your terms. Independence starts with mobility, and mobility starts with regular activity. So, let us dive into fun, easy, and downright enjoyable ways to stay active and independent.

Dance Like No One's Watching (Because No One Is)

Imagine this: your favorite song comes on. What do you do? Tap your foot? Nod your head? How about going full-on dance mode? Dancing is not just a ticket to fun—it is a stealth workout that improves balance, coordination, and cardio health. Whether it is a solo boogie in the living room or a salsa class at the local community center, dancing keeps you light on your feet and ready to take on the world.

Not into dance parties? No problem. Tai chi and yoga offer a slower, more meditative way to build strength and flexibility. Tai chi, often called "meditation in motion," helps you stay calm, centered, and stable. Yoga? It is like giving your body a hug, stretching your muscles while strengthening them. Bonus: both are great for your posture, so you will look and feel taller (hello, confidence boost!).

Walk This Way—Literally

Walking is the superhero of physical activity—no cape required. It is free, does not need fancy equipment, and can be done almost anywhere. Plus, it is not just about burning calories; it is about keeping your joints, muscles, and heart in top shape.

Start small. A stroll around the block or a quick walk to the park is a great beginning. Set goals, but keep them realistic—think steps, not marathons. And make it fun! Walk with a buddy, your grandkids, or even your dog. Got no dog? Borrow your neighbour's—they will thank you!

Pro tip: Spice up your walks. Explore a new trail, listen to an engaging podcast, or turn your stroll into a photo scavenger hunt. Walking is not just about the destination; it is about the journey—and the snacks waiting at the end (healthy ones, of course).

Lift, Push, and Pull—The Power of Strength Training

Before you roll your eyes at the idea of strength training, let us clear up a myth: it is not just for bodybuilders or gym rats. Even light weights or resistance bands can work wonders for your muscles, keeping them strong and ready to support you.

Cannot make it to the gym? No sweat. Your home is full of gym equipment in disguise. Soup cans become dumbbells, a sturdy chair transforms into a squat assistant, and your countertop? Perfect for push-ups! Start with easy moves and gradually increase the challenge. You will not only feel stronger but also find everyday tasks—like carrying groceries or getting up from a chair—a lot easier. And here is a bonus: strength training can help prevent falls. Strong muscles mean better balance and stability, and that is a game-changer when it comes to staying independent.

Balance: The Unsung Hero of Independence

Speaking of falls, let us talk balance. It is not just about staying upright—it is about confidence. Knowing you can move without wobbling or toppling is empowering.

Simple balance exercises can make a big difference. Try standing on one leg while brushing your teeth. Too easy? Close your eyes! (But maybe not with a toothbrush in hand—safety first.) Other great options include heel-to-toe walking or balancing on a foam pad. Do not overlook activities like Pilates or tai chi, which naturally improve balance and coordination. And remember, the key is consistency. A few minutes a day can keep the doctor—and the floor—away.

Keep Your Mind on Its Toes

Staying active is not just about your body—your brain needs exercise, too. Mental sharpness is crucial for independence, and the good news is that working your brain can be as fun as it is effective.

Love puzzles? Dive into crosswords, Sudoku, or jigsaw puzzles. Prefer something more interactive? Try board games or trivia nights with friends. And if you are feeling ambitious, why not learn a new skill? Pick up the ukulele, start painting, or even tackle a new language.

Technology can be your ally here. Brain-training apps, virtual chess games, or online courses make it easy to keep your mind engaged. Remember, a curious mind is a healthy mind—and it is never too late to learn something new.

Make It Social: The Secret Ingredient

Here is the thing: staying active does not have to be a solo mission. In fact, it is more fun (and often easier) when you involve others. Join a walking group, sign up for a dance class, or find a workout buddy. The accountability helps, but so does the camaraderie.

Socializing itself is a form of mental and emotional exercise. Loneliness can weigh on your heart, so keep your social calendar as active as your workout routine. Whether it is coffee dates, community events, or volunteering, staying connected keeps you engaged with the world —and that is a big part of staying independent. Staying active and independent is not about ticking off a checklist or following a strict routine. It is about finding what works for you and making it a joyful part of your life. Whether you are dancing in your living room, walking your neighborhood trails, or mastering a new skill, every little bit adds up. So, lace up your shoes, turn up the music, and embrace a life full of movement, laughter, and independence.

15.3 Planning For Long-Term Health

Let us be honest: thinking about the future, especially when it comes to health, is not exactly the stuff of daydreams. But here is the truth—future you will thank present you for taking a little time now to plan ahead. Consider this chapter your friendly tap on the shoulder to get things in order so you can glide through your golden years with grace, independence, and a whole lot of heart health.

Prevention: Your Secret Superpower

Think of prevention as your superhero cape—it is not flashy, but it saves the day. The most heroic thing you can do for your health? Keep up with regular check-ups. Annual physicals might sound about as exciting as waiting in line at the DMV, but they are worth every minute.

Your doctor is like a detective. They can spot those sneaky signs of trouble, like high blood pressure or cholesterol that is creeping up, long before you notice them. And trust me, catching these early is much easier (and less stressful) than dealing with the fallout later. Got high blood pressure? Treating it now protects your heart, your brain, and even your kidneys from unnecessary drama down the line. Do not wait until something feels off to schedule an appointment. Be proactive. Think of it as giving your heart a tune-up—no one wants to deal with a breakdown on the highway of life.

Nutrition: More Than Just Kale

Healthy eating is not about kale smoothies and quinoa bowls every day (though if you love those, more power to you). It is about balance, flavor, and making food your ally in long-term health.

Here is the deal: your heart loves good fats (like those in avocados, nuts, and olive oil), lean proteins, and fiber-rich carbs. But your taste buds? They love pizza and chocolate cake. So how do you keep everyone happy? Moderation.

Instead of swearing off your favorite foods, try making small swaps. Love pasta? Go half-and-half with whole wheat noodles. Craving something sweet? Pair a square of dark chocolate with fresh berries. Meal planning is your secret weapon here. Spend an hour on Sunday whipping up a big pot of vegetable soup or roasting a batch of chicken and veggies. Boom—you have got healthy meals ready to go when hunger strikes. Spices are another game-changer. Who said healthy food has to be boring? Add turmeric to your rice, paprika to your chicken, or cinnamon to your oatmeal. Your taste buds will thank you, and so will your heart.

Your Support Network: Build It Before You Need It

No one climbs a mountain alone, and the mountain of aging is no exception. Having a solid support system is not just nice; it is essential. So, who is in your corner?

Family is a great starting point, but do not stop there. Friends, neighbors, and even community groups can play a huge role. If you are not already connected to local resources, now is the time to start. Whether it is a walking group, a book club, or a church community, having people to lean on can make all the difference. And let us not forget the professionals. Your doctor, a good physiotherapist, and maybe even a nutritionist can be part of your dream team. These folks are like the pit crew for your race car—they keep you running smoothly. Most importantly, do not be afraid to ask for help. Need someone to grab groceries when you are feeling under the weather? Say so. Want company for a doctor's visit? Invite a friend. People want to help—they just need to know how.

Your Home: Safety Meets Comfort

Take a good look around your home. Is it ready to support you in the long run? If not, a few small tweaks can make a big difference.

Start with the bathroom—it is the most common place for accidents. Installing grab bars near the toilet and shower can prevent slips and give you peace of mind. Non-slip mats are another must-have. Lighting is another easy win. Brighten up dark hallways and add nightlights to help you navigate safely during those midnight trips to the fridge (or, let us be honest, the bathroom). Think about your kitchen, too. Are your everyday items within easy reach, or do you need to perform a mini-Cirque du Soleil routine to grab a plate? Reorganizing your space can make life a lot easier—and safer. If you are feeling fancy, consider tech upgrades like smart lights or voice-activated assistants. Who would not want to tell Alexa to turn off the lights without leaving the couch?

Do not Forget to Plan for Joy

Here is a little secret: planning for your health is not just about avoiding frailty or heart problems—it is about making room for joy. What is the point of living longer if you are not enjoying the ride?

Start by thinking about what lights you up. Is it painting, gardening, or learning to play the guitar? Maybe it is traveling to new places or revisiting old favourites. Whatever it is, be available for it. Your passions are not just good for your soul—they are good for your heart, too. Volunteering is another way to keep your heart happy. Helping others not only feels good, but it also keeps you active and connected to your community. Plus, it is a great way to meet like-minded people who share your interests. And let us not forget laughter. Watch that silly sitcom, swap dad jokes with your grandkids, or call up an old friend for a trip down memory lane. Laughter really is the best medicine—and it is free!

So, to sum up, preventing frailty and protecting your heart is not about living a life of restrictions; it is about making smart, joyful choices that add up over time. It is about saying yes to regular check-ups, no to chronic stress, and absolutely to chocolate (in moderation). From building a support network to creating a home that is safe and comfortable, each step you take today sets the stage for a healthier, happier tomorrow. So, go ahead—dance in the kitchen, laugh with your friends, and savor every bite of that heart-healthy meal. Future you is going to love the life you are building right now.

CHAPTER 16: FRAILTY AND HEART ATTACK

16.1 Rehabilitation And Recovery In Frail Patients

Recovering from a heart attack is not just about patching up your heart—it is about rebuilding your whole self. Cardiac rehabilitation helps older patients recover better after a heart attack. Their recovery is affected not just by the heart problem but also by other health issues and overall frailty (125). For frail patients, this can feel like climbing a mountain with a backpack full of bricks. But here is the good news: you do not have to sprint to the top on day one. Recovery is more like tending to a garden—it takes the right tools, some tender care, and a little patience. The journey can be tough, but with the right mindset and support, it is absolutely doable. Let us dig in.

Start Slow, Build Steady

The first few days after a heart attack might feel like someone hit your body's pause button. Everything seems harder—getting out of bed, taking a few steps, even holding a fork. Do not worry; this is normal. Think of it as the warm-up before a big game. You are not expected to run laps right now—just show up and stretch.

Step by Step

Imagine your heart as a worker returning to the job after a long break. It is eager but rusty and overloading it could spell trouble. Start with small movements: sitting up, dangling your legs off the bed, or shuffling a few steps with assistance. Each tiny action is a big win.

Why Rest Is not Always Best

It might sound counterintuitive, but lying in bed all day is not doing you any favors. Prolonged rest can weaken your muscles faster than you would believe. Even light activity—wiggling your toes, stretching your arms—keeps your body from falling into a deeper slump.

Celebrate the Little Things

Did you stand up without help today? Managed to shuffle to the bathroom on your own? These might seem like small achievements, but they are actually huge milestones in the grand scheme of recovery. Treat them like winning a gold medal—they are steps in the right direction.

Your Rehab Team: The Dream Squad

Rehabilitation is not a solo sport; it is a team effort. And lucky for you, your team is made up of some pretty awesome players. Picture them as the pit crew for your body, working tirelessly behind the scenes to make sure you are ready to hit the road again.

Who is on Your Team?

Doctors: They are the captains of the ship, steering your recovery in the right direction. They will monitor your progress and tweak the plan as needed.

Physiotherapists (PTs): PTs are like personal trainers, but gentler. They will guide you through exercises to rebuild strength, balance, and mobility.

Occupational therapists (OTs): OTs play a crucial role in cardiac rehabilitation by helping patients recover and improve their quality of life after a heart attack or other cardiac events. OTs evaluate patients' physical, cognitive, and emotional abilities to create personalized rehabilitation plans. They assist patients in regaining the ability to perform daily tasks such as dressing, bathing, and cooking.

Dietitians: Food is fuel, and dietitians are your go-to experts for crafting meals that nourish without overwhelming your recovering heart.

Nurses: The unsung heroes of healthcare, nurses are there to answer questions, address concerns, and keep you comfortable.

How to Work with Your Team

Be honest about how you are feeling—good, bad, or ugly. If an exercise hurts, say so. If you are feeling anxious, speak up. This is not the time to tough it out; your team cannot help if they do not know what is going on.

Set Small Goals

When you are frail, the idea of "getting back to normal" can feel like an impossible dream. But here is the thing: recovery is not about overnight transformation. It is about chipping away at the mountain one tiny step at a time.

The Magic of Micro-Goals

Instead of aiming to climb stairs or jog around the block, set goals you can achieve in a day or two. Can you sit up without help? Walk to the window? Cook a light meal? Each small win builds momentum and confidence.

Track Your Progress

Keep a journal or checklist of your daily achievements. Seeing your progress on paper—no matter how small—can be incredibly motivating. Plus, it gives you a reason to high-five yourself every evening.

Reward Yourself

Did you achieve a goal? Celebrate! Watch your favorite show, enjoy a piece of dark chocolate, or spend a few extra minutes chatting with a friend. Rewards keep you motivated and make the journey a little more fun.

The Frailty-Hospital Loop

Let us talk about one of recovery's biggest challenges: the frailty-hospital loop. Long hospital stays can sap your strength faster than a smartphone battery on low power mode. For frail patients, this creates a vicious cycle—frailty leads to longer stays, which worsen frailty, which leads to more health issues.

Why Early Rehab Matters

The sooner you start rehab, the better your chances of breaking this loop. Gentle movement prevents muscle atrophy, keeps your circulation humming, and helps your body bounce back faster.

Home Sweet Home

Getting discharged does not mean the end of the journey. In fact, it is just the beginning. Continuing rehab at home—with guidance from your dream squad—is crucial for maintaining the progress you have made.

Stay Positive

It is easy to feel overwhelmed but remember: every journey has its setbacks. Do not let a bad day discourage you. Keep your focus on the bigger picture—a healthier, stronger you.

Recovering from a heart attack while managing frailty is not easy, but it is far from impossible. With the right tools, the right team, and a hefty dose of patience, you can rebuild your strength, reclaim your independence, and start living life to the fullest again. One step at a time, you have got this.

16.2 Steps To Regain Strength And Confidence

Regaining strength after a heart attack is not about rushing to the finish line; it is about building a strong, sturdy house one brick at a time. Your foundation is basic mobility—getting your body back in motion. From there, you can add layers like balance, stamina, and, perhaps most importantly, confidence. Yes, confidence. It is just as essential as physical strength, and it grows with each small victory. Let us break it down into manageable, engaging, and even enjoyable steps.

Start with the Core: Strengthening Basics

Forget the idea that recovery means hitting the gym hard. For frail patients, less is more. Start with activities you can do at home. Use what is around you: a sturdy chair, soup cans, or even your own body weight. Here are some exercises that do not require spandex or dumbbells:

Chair Exercises: Sit, stand, repeat. It is simple but powerful. Standing up from a chair without using your hands strengthens your legs and boosts balance.

Soup Can Lifts: Grab those cans of tomato soup sitting in your pantry. They make great light weights for arm exercises.

Stretch It Out: Gentle stretches for your legs, arms, and back improve flexibility and reduce stiffness. Start with a reach-for-the-sky motion, and you will feel a little taller—if not prouder.

Hand Squeezes: A stress ball or a rolled-up sock can be squeezed to strengthen your grip. It is oddly satisfying and surprisingly effective.

Progress at your own pace. You are not training for a marathon; you are retraining your body to handle daily life with ease.

Eat Like a Champion

Your recovery does not just happen on the exercise mat—it starts on your plate. Nutrition is your secret weapon for regaining strength. Think of your meals as a construction crew working on your "house of recovery." Here is the menu for a champion:

Protein Power: Eggs, beans, chicken, tofu, and fish are like bricks for building muscle. Aim to include a protein source in every meal.

Micronutrient Magic: Fruits, veggies, and whole grains provide the vitamins and minerals your body craves. Leafy greens like spinach are packed with iron, which helps combat fatigue.

Hydration Nation: Even mild dehydration can make you feel sluggish and weak. Keep a water bottle handy, and sip throughout the day. (Tip: Add a slice of lemon for a refreshing twist.)

Snack Smart: Nuts, yogurt, or a piece of fruit are perfect pick-me-ups. Avoid the temptation of sugary snacks—they are like fireworks: a quick burst of energy followed by a big crash.

Eating well is not about strict rules; it is about nourishing your body with foods that help you feel strong and energized.

Mind Over Matter

Let us be real: recovery is not just physical. Your brain and emotions play a huge role. After a heart attack, fear and frustration can sneak in like uninvited guests. Here is how to kick them out and invite positivity instead:

Meditation Moments: Spend 5–10 minutes a day focusing on your breath. It calms your mind and lowers stress, which is great for your heart.

Find Your Happy Place: Whether it is gardening, knitting, or watching funny videos of cats, doing something you love can lift your spirits. Laughter, after all, is great medicine.

Set Small Wins: Big goals can feel overwhelming. Instead, focus on achievable steps like walking to the mailbox or preparing a simple meal. Each win builds confidence.

Talk It Out: Share your thoughts with someone you trust. Bottling up emotions is like shaking a soda can—it is bound to explode at some point.

Remember, your mindset can either be your greatest ally or your biggest hurdle. Choose to be your own cheerleader.

Buddy System Bonus

Recovery is a team sport. Having someone by your side—whether it is a friend, family member, or even a furry companion—makes the journey feel less daunting.

Accountability Partner: A friend who checks in on your progress can keep you motivated. Bonus points if they join you for walks or exercise sessions.

Support Groups: Sometimes, sharing your journey with others in the same boat can be incredibly comforting. Look for local or online groups for heart attack survivors.

Pet Power: Pets are natural motivators. Dogs make great walking buddies, while cats can be excellent listeners (even if they look unimpressed).

Family Fun: Turn recovery into quality family time. Play light games, cook healthy meals together, or simply share a laugh over a good movie.

Companionship is not just about having someone to talk to; it is about feeling connected and supported. And let us face it—everything is better with a little company.

Recovery is a journey of rediscovery. It is about finding strength in small moments and building confidence step by step. There is no rush and no competition—just you, steadily rebuilding your house of health with care, patience, and maybe even a little humour. Because let us face it: a good laugh might not tone your abs, but it sure makes the process a lot more fun.

16.3 Avoiding Complications After A Cardiac Event

Recovering from a heart attack is like navigating a winding road—you have made it past the steepest hill, but a wrong turn could land you in a ditch. Complications can sneak up like potholes, but with the right strategies, you will cruise through recovery safely. Let us dive into how you can stay on track and out of trouble.

Watch for Warning Signs

Your body is like a smoke alarm—it will not stay quiet if something is wrong. Chest pain, dizziness, swelling, or shortness of breath are not just random glitches. They are your body's SOS signals.

When to Raise the Alarm

Sure, we all have off days, but if your chest feels like a weight is pressing down, your feet look puffier than marshmallows, or you are getting lightheaded every time you stand up, it is time to call your doctor—or an ambulance. Do not be a hero; early intervention saves lives.

The Silent Warnings

Not every warning is obvious. Fatigue that does not quit or unusual sweating could be sneaky signs of trouble. Think of them as whispers before the shout—listen to your body.

Keep a Symptom Diary

A diary is not just for teenage crushes. Jotting down symptoms can help your doctor connect the dots. It is like creating a map of your health—one that helps steer you back to safety if complications arise.

Medication: Your Silent Partner

Ah, medications. Not glamorous, not fun, but absolutely essential. Think of them as the backstage crew making sure your body performs its best.

Set It, Do not Forget It

Consistency is key. Take your pills like clockwork—because skipping doses is not just rebellious; it is dangerous. If you struggle to remember, set reminders on your phone, use a pill organizer, or tie it to your daily coffee ritual.

Know What You are Taking

Ever heard of "know your enemy"? Well, know your ally too! Learn what each medication does. That way, you will understand why that tiny aspirin or beta-blocker is doing big things for your heart.

Side Effects Are not Deal-Breakers

Feeling a little off? Some side effects might fade as your body adjusts. But if they are making you miserable, do not ghost your meds—talk to your doctor. There is often a workaround.

Avoid DIY Dosing

Missed a dose? Resist the urge to double up. Ask your nurse first. Medicine is not like calories—there is no "make-up day." Follow your doctor's orders to the letter; they have got your back.

Keep Moving, But Do not Overdo It

Movement is medicine, but too much can be poison. Think of your recovery as a game of Goldilocks—you need "just right" activity to keep your heart and body happy.

Start with Baby Steps

Begin with simple activities. A slow walk around the living room might not feel like much, but for your heart, it is a celebration. Gradually increase the intensity as you feel stronger.

Listen to Your Body

Pushing yourself too hard can backfire. If you feel short of breath, overly fatigued, or in pain, it is your body's way of saying, "Whoa, buddy. Take it easy."

Build Balance and Strength

Beyond walking, try gentle exercises like yoga or tai chi. These activities improve balance and strength while keeping your heart rate steady. Plus, they are great for calming your mind—double win!

Consult Your Rehab Team

Before starting any exercise, check with your rehab team. They will tailor a program that is safe and effective for you. No guessing games here—let the pros guide you.

Stay Connected

Isolation is not just lonely—it is downright risky. Staying socially active can improve your mood, keep you motivated, and even boost your physical recovery.

The Power of a Good Chat

Whether it is a phone call with your grandkids or a coffee date with a neighbour, staying socially engaged works wonders for your recovery. Laughter might not fix a leaky heart valve, but it can mend your spirit.

Join a Support Group

You are not alone in this journey. A cardiac rehab group or local senior club can introduce you to people who have been in your shoes. Sharing stories and tips makes the path feel less daunting.

Family and Friends: Your Recovery Cheerleaders

Lean on your loved ones for help and encouragement. Whether they are fetching groceries or just listening to you vent, their support can make a world of difference.

Technology to the Rescue

If getting out is tough, let tech be your lifeline. Video calls, online forums, or even social media can help you stay connected. Virtual hugs count too!

Recovering after a heart attack while managing frailty is no small feat, but you have got this. Remember, avoiding complications is not about being perfect—it is about staying alert, following your plan, and celebrating progress, no matter how small. Keep an eye on those warning signs, embrace your meds, move with purpose, and surround yourself with love and support. With these strategies, you are not just surviving—you are thriving. Keep going, one heart-healthy step at a time.

CHAPTER 17: FRAILTY AND SURGERY

Surgery is no walk in the park, even for the sprightly among us. But when frailty steps into the mix, things get a tad more complicated. Think of it like adding a wobbly wheel to a cart you are trying to push uphill—it can still be done, but with a bit more care and some clever planning. Let us explore how frailty intersects with cardiac procedures, how to prepare for surgery when frail, and what challenges might pop up after the operation (126).

17.1 Frailty And Cardiac Procedures

Cardiac procedures can be lifesavers—literally. From bypass surgeries to valve repairs, they keep the heart ticking. But for frail individuals, these procedures come with added risks. Why? Because frailty's baggage includes reduced strength, slower recovery, and a body that is less able to bounce back from big stressors. Surgery is one such stressor.

The Risky Business of Surgery

When a frail person undergoes surgery, it is like asking a tired marathon runner to sprint another mile. They can do it, but not without potentially hitting some hurdles. These hurdles include a greater likelihood of complications like infections, longer hospital stays, or even needing more help to get back to daily life afterward.

Common Cardiac Procedures and Frailty's Role

Let us break it down:

Bypass Surgery: A lifesaver for blocked arteries but can feel like a marathon for the body. Frailty can make recovery slower, and the risk of post-surgery issues like confusion or weakness is higher.

Valve Replacements: Whether traditional or minimally invasive, frail individuals may face higher risks of complications like infections or longer recovery times.

Pacemaker Implantation: Usually a smaller procedure, but frailty can still slow healing and complicate post-op care.

What Can Be Done?

Doctors are getting pretty good at spotting frailty before surgery. They will weigh the risks and benefits and might suggest alternatives if the risks are sky-high. Minimally invasive procedures are often a great choice for frail patients—think of it as replacing a jackhammer with a gentle tap.

17.2 Preparing For Surgery When Frail

Preparation is key—kind of like packing for a big trip. If you are frail, prepping for surgery means more than just showing up at the hospital. It is about building strength, managing stress, and getting your body as ready as possible to tackle the challenge ahead.

Strengthening for Surgery

Think of this as pre-surgery boot camp. No, you will not need to do push-ups or run laps, but even small steps can make a big difference:

Eat Up: A nutrient-rich diet—full of protein and essential vitamins—can give your body the tools it needs to heal better and faster.

Move It: Gentle exercises like walking or light strength training can boost your stamina and muscle mass, making recovery smoother.

Quit the Bad Stuff: If you smoke or drink heavily, now is the time to cut back. Your body will thank you during recovery.

Mental Prep Matters Too

Surgery can be stressful. Frailty's emotional companions, like anxiety or depression, can make it feel even more daunting. Talking to a counsellor, meditating, or even just chatting with friends and family can ease the mental load.

Rally the Troops

Let us face it, surgery is not a solo journey. Having a solid support system—family, friends, or caregivers—can make a world of difference. They can help you get to appointments, manage medications, and cheer you on through recovery.

17.3 Post-Surgical Challenges And Recovery

Once the surgery is done, the real work begins. For frail individuals, the post-op period can feel like climbing a mountain—but with the right tools and team, that climb is totally doable.

Common Challenges

Slow Recovery: Healing takes longer for frail folks, so patience is key.

Confusion or Delirium: Post-surgery brain fog is common and can be unsettling. It is usually temporary but might need medical attention (127).

Weakness and Fatigue: Expect to feel wiped out. Rest and gradual activity are the name of the game.

Building Back Better

Physical Therapy: Your new best friend. Therapists can guide you through exercises to regain strength and mobility.

Nutritional Support: Keep those nutrients coming. Protein shakes, balanced meals, and hydration are your allies.

Emotional Recovery: Post-surgery blues are a thing. Do not hesitate to seek support if you are feeling down.

The Importance of Follow-Ups

Recovery does not end when you leave the hospital. Regular check-ins with your healthcare team can catch issues early and keep you on the right track.

Setting Realistic Goals

Rome was not built in a day, and neither is a full recovery. Celebrate small wins, whether it is walking a few steps more than yesterday or finally being able to enjoy your favorite meal again. However, we will not delve into deeper on this technical issues and that is out of the scope of this book.

CHAPTER 18: CAREGIVING FOR FRAIL ADULTS

18.1 How To Support A Frail Loved One

Caring for someone who is frail and dealing with heart disease (128-130) is no small feat. It is a little like juggling flaming torches while riding a unicycle – challenging, sure, but not impossible! The secret is finding balance, staying prepared, and giving yourself some grace along the way.

First things first: understand their needs. Frailty is not just about being a bit tired; it is a whole mix of physical, emotional, and social challenges. Heart disease adds its complications, making daily tasks more demanding and sometimes downright exhausting for your loved one. So, be observant. Notice when they are struggling to get out of bed or when their mood seems off. Small changes can be clues to bigger issues.

Communication is key. Ask questions like, "What can I do to make your day easier?" or "How are you feeling today?" And really listen to the answers. Sometimes, what they need most is a cup of tea and a patient ear.

Physical support might involve helping with mobility, managing medications, or assisting with doctor's appointments. Do not shy away from asking the healthcare team for tips. Many hospitals and clinics offer training sessions or have resources to teach caregivers how to handle these tasks safely. Pro tip: Learn how to use a pill organizer – it will save you and your loved one from countless, "Did you take your meds?" conversations.

Emotional support is just as important. Encourage hobbies or social activities, even if it is something as simple as a phone call with an old friend. Loneliness can sneak in, and that is a heavy burden to bear.

Finally, do not forget about your own well-being. You cannot pour from an empty cup, so schedule regular breaks, lean on your support network, and give yourself permission to have bad days. After all, caregiving is not a sprint; it is a marathon, and pacing yourself is necessary.

18.2 Balancing Heart Health And Quality Of Life

Now here is the kicker: how do you keep your loved one's heart ticking along nicely while ensuring they still get to enjoy life? Because let us face it, nobody wants to trade chocolate cake for celery sticks forever. The trick is finding that sweet spot between heart health and happiness.

Start with diet. Yes, heart-healthy eating matters, but it does not have to mean endless plates of kale. Work with a dietitian to create meals that are nutritious and delicious. Maybe swap fried chicken for baked salmon or sneak some avocado onto their toast. Keep treats in the mix, too – moderation is your best friend.

Next up, movement. Frailty does not mean they are stuck on the couch 24/7. Gentle activities like walking, chair yoga, or even light gardening can work wonders for both physical and mental health. Just make sure the exercise is tailored to their abilities. Think "slow and steady" rather than "Let's run a marathon!"

Then there's medication management. Heart disease often comes with a long list of prescriptions, which can feel like a full-time job to keep track of. Double-check dosing schedules, watch for side effects, and do not hesitate to ask the pharmacist questions. A simple tip? Set reminders on your phone or use a color-coded chart.

Quality of life is about more than just staying physically well. It is also about finding joy in the little things. Help them savor their favorite hobbies, whether it is knitting, crossword puzzles, or watching old sitcoms. And if they are feeling adventurous, try something new together – a virtual cooking class, perhaps, or a drive to a scenic spot.

Most importantly, keep the focus on what is meaningful to them. Whether it is celebrating family milestones, enjoying a good meal, or simply having a heart-to-heart conversation, these moments are the true heartbeats of life.

18.3 Resources For Caregivers

Being a caregiver can feel like you are stranded on a deserted island with nothing but a Swiss Army knife and a half-charged phone. But here is the good news: you are not alone. There are resources out there to help you navigate this journey, and tapping into them can make all the difference.

Let us start with the basics: support groups. Whether in-person or online, these groups offer a safe space to vent, share tips, and connect with others who truly get it. Sometimes, just hearing, "I've been there too," can lift a huge weight off your shoulders.

Professional services are another lifeline. Home health aides, visiting nurses, or meal delivery programs can take some of the pressure off your plate. Many communities also have adult day care centers where your loved one can spend a few hours socializing while you catch up on errands or simply take a breather.

Educational resources are invaluable. Organizations like Heart Association or local geriatric societies often provide workshops, webinars, and guides on everything from managing medications to coping with caregiver stress. You might even find a few helpful apps to streamline things like appointment scheduling or symptom tracking.

Financial and legal assistance can be a game-changer. If you are feeling overwhelmed by medical bills or unsure about insurance options, reach out to social workers or financial counsellors. They are pros at untangling red tape and finding solutions.

Lastly, do not underestimate the power of self-care. Many caregiver support programs offer respite services, so you can take a well-deserved break. Whether it is a spa day, a coffee with friends, or just an uninterrupted nap, recharging your batteries is essential.

Remember, asking for help is not a sign of weakness; it is a strategy for success. By leaning on these resources, you are not only helping your loved one but also ensuring you can continue to be their rock. Caregiving is tough, but with the right tools and a little humour, you have got this!

CHAPTER 19: INNOVATIONS IN FRAILTY MANAGEMENT

19.1 How To Monitor Frailty

The Tech Revolution: Gadgets That Keep an Eye on You

Once upon a time, doctors relied on a firm handshake and a bit of guesswork to assess frailty. Today, we have swapped out guesswork for gadgets. From wearable fitness trackers to high-tech smart scales, innovation has opened up new ways to monitor frailty like never before (131). These devices do not just count steps—they measure heart rate, muscle activity, sleep quality, and even how well you balance on one foot. Yes, your Fitbit might know you are wobbly before you do!

But here is the real magic: these gadgets collect data over time. Think of it as a diary of your health, minus the effort of actually keeping a diary. They can spot trends, like a gradual slowing of your walk or nights of restless sleep, which could hint at frailty brewing under the surface. And the best part? Many devices are designed to blend seamlessly into your life, so you can track your health while binge-watching your favorite series.

Still, it is not all smooth sailing. These gadgets come with batteries that seem allergic to lasting, and they can get a little judgy if you skip a walk (or two). But paired with professional medical advice, they are an excellent way to keep tabs on how your body is holding up (132).

The Art of Observation: What Your Everyday Moves Reveal

Not every frailty test needs a lab coat or a gadget. In fact, some of the best tools for spotting frailty are the things you do daily—like getting out of bed, climbing stairs, or lifting a grocery bag. These "everyday tasks" are secretly health checks in disguise. Struggling to open that stubborn pickle jar? It might mean more than you think.

Doctors use simple tests like the Timed Up and Go (TUG)—basically, they time how quickly you can stand, walk a short distance, and sit back down. It is simple, but it works. Why? Because frailty often sneaks up in subtle ways. Slower movements, hesitation, or a loss of confidence in your stride can all be clues. But there are a wide ranges of frailty assessment tools used by different health professionals in different settings (66).

So, keep an eye on how you are moving through the world. Can you keep up with your grandkids during a game of tag? (Okay, maybe not entirely fair, but you get the idea.) Spotting small changes early means you can act before frailty becomes a bigger challenge.

The Numbers Game: Blood Tests, Biomarkers, and Beyond

Your blood has secrets, and it is not shy about spilling them. From inflammation levels to nutrient deficiencies, a simple blood test can reveal if your body is running out of steam. Scientists are even developing biomarkers—fancy biological indicators—to detect frailty with more precision than ever before (133-135). Let us break it down: certain proteins and hormones can hint at muscle loss or fatigue, while vitamin D and iron levels might point to nutritional gaps. These tests are not just diagnostic—they are a way to tailor solutions to your specific needs. Think of it as a health blueprint, helping your doctor build a plan that is just right for you.

But remember, numbers do not tell the whole story. You are more than your lab results! Pair these tests with a chat about how you are feeling and moving. After all, science works best when combined with your lived experience.

The Future Is AI: Robots and Algorithms to the Rescue

Cue the futuristic soundtrack—artificial intelligence (AI) is entering the frailty arena (136, 137). Picture this: a robot in your living room measuring your gait speed or analyzing the tone of your voice for signs of fatigue. Or an app that predicts your frailty risk based on your daily activities, diet, and even how often you call your family.

AI is also transforming medical consultations. Algorithms can analyze mountains of data from your electronic health records to flag early signs of frailty. It is like having a health detective working behind the scenes, spotting patterns even the sharpest doctor might miss.

Of course, there are hiccups. Technology is not perfect, and it is only as good as the data it is fed (136). But as AI learns and improves, it promises to revolutionize how we monitor frailty, making it faster, more accurate, and more personalized.

Keeping It Real: What You Can Do at Home

Here is the good news: you do not need to wait for the next big innovation to start monitoring frailty. Some of the best tools are already at your fingertips. Try this quick test: stand on one leg and time yourself. If you wobble before 10 seconds, it might be time to work on balance. Or take the stairs instead of the elevator and notice how you feel—winded, steady, or somewhere in between? Journaling your daily energy levels, sleep, and diet is another powerful (and low-tech) way to track changes. You do not need to draft an essay—a few notes here and there can provide valuable insights over time. And remember, this is not about catching frailty —it is about staying ahead of it. Monitoring means you can take small, manageable steps to stay strong and independent, whether it is tweaking your diet, trying a new exercise, or just taking a little extra time to rest.

Frailty might feel like a big, scary word, but monitoring it does not have to be intimidating. With tools ranging from high-tech gadgets to simple observations, there are plenty of ways to keep tabs on your health. And the sooner you start paying attention, the more options you have to stay one step ahead—literally and figuratively.

19.2 Emerging Treatments And Technologies

Imagine a world where diagnosing frailty is as easy as snapping your fingers. Well, we are not quite there yet, but the innovations in this field are pretty exciting! Researchers and tech wizards are working overtime to bring us cutting-edge solutions that could revolutionize frailty care.

Wearable devices, like smartwatches, are leading the charge (131). These gadgets can track steps, heart rate, and even subtle changes in walking patterns. Some advanced models can predict the risk of falls before they happen—it is like having a fortune teller on your wrist (138)! Then there are apps designed to measure grip strength or detect voice changes that may signal cognitive decline. Who knew your phone could double as a mini health lab?

Robotics is another game-changer (139). Robotic exoskeletons might sound like something out of a sci-fi movie, but they are already helping people regain mobility (140). Picture a lightweight suit that supports their muscles and joints, making it easier to walk or even climb stairs. And let us not forget artificial intelligence. AI algorithms can analyze medical records, pinpoint frailty risks, and suggest personalized treatment plans faster than you can say "algorithm."

On the treatment front, scientists are exploring novel therapies (141). One promising avenue is the use of myostatin inhibitors to promote muscle growth (141). Imagine turning back the clock on muscle weakness! And regenerative medicine, including stem cell therapy, could help repair damaged tissues and improve overall function (142, 143). While these breakthroughs are still in the experimental stage, they are a beacon of hope for many.

19.3 The Role Of Preventive Medicine

Getting older comes with unavoidable changes to the body, like muscle loss (sarcopenia), bone thinning (osteoporosis), and frailty. Besides staying active and eating well, so far there are no effective treatments to stop these age-related changes (142). However, an ounce of prevention is worth a pound of cure, or in this case, a whole lot of strength and vitality. Preventive medicine is not just about avoiding illnesses; it is about building resilience, so frailty does not stand a chance.

Regular check-ups are your first line of defense. They are like taking your car for servicing —catching small issues before they turn into costly repairs. Screenings for bone density, muscle strength, and cognitive function can help spot early signs of frailty. And let us not forget vaccines. Staying up to date on flu and pneumonia shots can prevent infections that often lead to severe complications in frail individuals.

Physical activity is a cornerstone of prevention (141). No, you do not need to drag your loved one to a CrossFit class. Simple exercises, like walking, yoga, or resistance training with light weights, can strengthen muscles and improve balance. Even dancing around the living room counts—and it is way more fun!

Nutrition plays a starring role (141), too. Think of food as medicine. A diet rich in lean proteins, healthy fats, and colorful fruits and veggies can do wonders. Encourage hydration, too; dehydration is a sneaky frailty culprit. And if they are not big eaters, supplements might fill in the gaps, but always consult a doctor first.

Finally, *mental health* deserves a spotlight. Stress and depression can accelerate frailty, so promote relaxation techniques like mindfulness or meditation. Even a daily gratitude journal can help shift their mindset. Preventive medicine is not about waiting for a problem to knock on the door—it is about locking the door and tossing the key into the ocean.

CHAPTER 20: LIVING WITH FRAILTY AND HEART DISEASE

20.1 Redefining Success And Happiness

Living with frailty and heart disease can feel like a tightrope walk. You are balancing on a wire, trying to stay upright while life throws all sorts of challenges your way. But what if we told you that success does not always mean crossing the wire without a wobble? Sometimes, it is about embracing the wobbles and finding joy in the journey.

Success and happiness, when living with frailty and heart disease, often need a little rebranding. Instead of focusing on what you cannot do, start celebrating what you can. Maybe you cannot run a marathon (who really wants to, anyway?), but you can still enjoy a brisk walk in the park. Maybe lifting heavy groceries is out of the question, but arranging a family potluck means less stress and more bonding time. Redefining success means shifting your goals to fit your abilities—and taking pride in achieving them.

It is also about finding happiness in the small things. Ever noticed how a cup of tea tastes better when you are fully present in the moment? Or how a phone call with a loved one can brighten your day? These seemingly simple joys become the building blocks of a fulfilling life. So, trade those impossible expectations for realistic ones. Celebrate progress, no matter how small, and let your definition of success evolve with you.

20.2 Real-Life Stories Of Resilience

There is no better way to understand living well with frailty and heart disease than by hearing from people who have done it. Let us meet a few resilient warriors who have turned challenges into triumphs.

Take *Ms X*, for instance. At 72, she was diagnosed with frailty and coronary artery disease. It was a double whammy that left her reeling. But she decided to take charge. She joined a local support group, started a gentle yoga routine, and began meal prepping with her granddaughter every Sunday. Today, she swears by her "Three Ps": Positivity, Patience, and Protein (she loves her grilled salmon!). Her secret? Focus on what she calls her "Good Day Checklist"—simple tasks like stretching, reading a chapter of her favorite book, and calling a friend.

Then there's *Mr Y*, an 80-year-old retired teacher who has become the unofficial "frailty guru" of his neighborhood. He runs a gardening club where members not only grow tomatoes but also exchange tips on managing their health. His advice? "Frailty is not a life sentence; it is just a call to adapt." He is proof that resilience grows stronger with community.

These stories remind us that resilience does not mean ignoring the tough parts. It is about facing them head-on and finding ways to thrive despite the odds. Whether it is Ms X's yoga mat or Mr Y's gardening gloves, resilience comes in many forms. What is yours?

20.3 Practical Tips For Patients And Families

Living well with frailty and heart disease is not just about medical treatments or diet plans. It is about crafting a lifestyle that works for you and your loved ones. Here are some practical tips to make the journey smoother and more enjoyable:

Teamwork Makes the Dream Work: You are not in this alone. Build a team of cheerleaders —family, friends, healthcare providers, and even your pharmacist. They are there to support, encourage, and help you navigate challenges. Do not hesitate to delegate tasks or ask for help. Remember, teamwork turns the "me" in medicine into "we."

Move It, But Do not Lose It: Gentle exercise is a game-changer. Whether it is tai chi, a short stroll, or dancing to your favorite song in the kitchen, find ways to keep moving. Exercise does not just strengthen muscles; it lifts your mood and boosts your confidence.

Food is Fuel—Make It Count: Your plate is your power. Load it with colorful veggies, lean proteins, and heart-healthy fats. Experiment with easy-to-digest meals that pack a nutritional punch. And do not forget to stay hydrated. Pro tip: If plain water feels boring, add a splash of lemon or a few cucumber slices.

Mind Over Matter: Managing stress is crucial. Try mindfulness exercises, deep breathing, or even a hobby like knitting or painting. A calm mind leads to a healthier heart.

Keep Talking: Communication is the glue that holds everything together. Share your thoughts, fears, and needs with your loved ones. And do not shy away from discussing your condition openly with your doctor. Honest conversations lead to better care.

Celebrate Every Victory: Whether it is standing up without assistance or making it through a medical appointment, celebrate your wins. They are proof of your strength and determination.

Remember, living well with frailty and heart disease is not about perfection. It is about making the most of every moment and finding joy in the little things. With the right mindset and support, you can lead a fulfilling, happy life—wobbles and all.

ABBREVIATIONS

ACE: Angiotensin-Converting Enzyme

AI: Artificial Intelligence

ARB: Angiotensin Receptor Blockers

CBT: Cognitive Behavioral Therapy

CFS: Clinical Frailty Scale

CHD: Coronary Heart Disease

CKD: Chronic Kidney Disease

COPD: Chronic Obstructive Pulmonary Disease

CVD: Cardiovascular Disease

DIY: Do It Yourself

DM: Diabetes mellitus

DMV: Department of Motor Vehicles

DOAC: Direct Oral Anticoagulant

EFS: Edmonton Frail Scale

FFP: Fried Frailty Phenotype

FI: Frailty Index

GPS: Global Positioning System

HDL: High Density Cholesterol

HRT: Hormone Replacement Therapy

IHD: Ischaemic Heart Disease

LDL: Low Density Lipoprotein

MACE: Major Adverse Cardiovascular Events

MVP: Most Valuable Player

OT: Occupational Therapist

PT: Physical Therapist

R&R: Rest and Recreation

TLC: Tender Loving Care

TUG: Timed Up and Go

REFERENCES

1) Fried LP, Tangen CM, Walston J, Newman AB, Hirsch C, Gottdiener J. Frailty in older adults: evidence for a phenotype. J Gerontol A Biol Sci Med Sci. 2001; 56.

2) Badimon L, Padró T, Vilahur G. Atherosclerosis, platelets and thrombosis in acute ischaemic heart disease. Eur Heart J Acute Cardiovasc Care. 2012; 1 (1): 60-74.

3) Razo C, Welgan CA, Johnson CO, McLaughlin SA, Iannucci V, Rodgers A, et al. Effects of elevated systolic blood pressure on ischemic heart disease: a Burden of Proof study. Nature Medicine. 2022; 28 (10): 2056-65.

4) Varbo A, Benn M, Nordestgaard BG. Remnant cholesterol as a cause of ischemic heart disease: Evidence, definition, measurement, atherogenicity, high risk patients, and present and future treatment. Pharmacology & Therapeutics. 2014; 141 (3): 358-67.

5) Schwinger RHG. Pathophysiology of heart failure. Cardiovasc Diagn Ther. 2021; 11 (1): 263-76.

6) Hajar R. Genetics in Cardiovascular Disease. Heart Views. 2020; 21 (1): 55-6.

7) Veronese N. Frailty as Cardiovascular Risk Factor (and Vice Versa). Adv Exp Med Biol. 2020; 1216: 51-4.

8) Ferrucci L, Fabbri E. Inflammageing: chronic inflammation in ageing, cardiovascular disease, and frailty. Nat Rev Cardiol. 2018; 15 (9): 505-22.

9) Clarke DM, Currie KC. Depression, anxiety and their relationship with chronic diseases: a review of the epidemiology, risk and treatment evidence. Med J Aust. 2009; 190 (S7): S54-60.

10) Seino S, Nishi M, Murayama H, Narita M, Yokoyama Y, Nofuji Y, et al. Effects of a multifactorial intervention comprising resistance exercise, nutritional and psychosocial programs on frailty and functional health in community-dwelling older adults: A randomized, controlled, cross-over trial. Geriatrics & gerontology international. 2017; 17 (11): 2034-45.

11) Firth J, Gangwisch JE, Borisini A, Wootton RE, Mayer EA. Food and mood: how do diet and nutrition affect mental wellbeing? BMJ. 2020; 369: m2382.

12) Libby P. The changing landscape of atherosclerosis. Nature. 2021; 592 (7855): 524-33.

13) Richter D, Guasti L, Walker D, Lambrinou E, Lionis C, Abreu A, et al. Frailty in cardiology: definition, assessment and clinical implications for general cardiology. A consensus document of the Council for Cardiology Practice (CCP), Association for Acute Cardio Vascular Care (ACVC), Association of Cardiovascular Nursing and Allied Professions (ACNAP), European Association of Preventive Cardiology (EAPC), European Heart Rhythm Association (EHRA), Council on Valvular Heart Diseases (VHD), Council on Hypertension (CHT), Council of Cardio-Oncology (CCO), Working Group (WG) Aorta and Peripheral Vascular Diseases, WG e-Cardiology, WG Thrombosis, of the European Society of Cardiology, European Primary Care Cardiology Society (EPCCS). European Journal of Preventive Cardiology. 2021; 29 (1): 216-27.

14) James K, Jamil Y, Kumar M, Kwak MJ, Nanna MG, Qazi S, et al. Frailty and Cardiovascular Health. Journal of the American Heart Association. 2024; 13 (15): e031736.

15) Afilalo J. Frailty in Patients with Cardiovascular Disease: Why, When, and How to Measure. Current Cardiovascular Risk Reports. 2011; 5 (5): 467-72.

16) Paneni F, Diaz Cañestro C, Libby P, Lüscher TF, Camici GG. The Aging Cardiovascular System: Understanding It at the Cellular and Clinical Levels. Journal of the American College of Cardiology. 2017; 69 (15): 1952-67.

17) Kramer CK, Leitao CB. Laughter as medicine: A systematic review and meta-analysis of interventional studies evaluating the impact of spontaneous laughter on cortisol levels. PLOS ONE. 2023; 18 (5): e0286260.

18) Rippe JM. Lifestyle Strategies for Risk Factor Reduction, Prevention, and Treatment of Cardiovascular Disease. Am J Lifestyle Med. 2019; 13 (2): 204-12.

19) Soysal P, Arik F, Smith L, Jackson SE, Isik AT. Inflammation, Frailty and Cardiovascular Disease. Adv Exp Med Biol. 2020; 1216: 55-64.

20) Hossain MN, Lee J, Choi H, Kwak YS, Kim J. The impact of exercise on depression: how moving makes your brain and body feel better. Phys Act Nutr. 2024; 28 (2): 43-51.

21) Knezevic E, Nenic K, Milanovic V, Knezevic NN. The Role of Cortisol in Chronic Stress, Neurodegenerative Diseases, and Psychological Disorders. Cells. 2023; 12 (23): 2726.

22) Dimsdale JE. Psychological stress and cardiovascular disease. J Am Coll Cardiol. 2008; 51 (13): 1237-46.

23) National Center for Chronic Disease P, Health Promotion Office on S, Health. Reports of the Surgeon General. The Health Consequences of Smoking—50 Years of Progress: A Report of the Surgeon General. Atlanta (GA): Centers for Disease Control and Prevention (US); 2014.

24) Kondo T, Nakano Y, Adachi S, Murohara T. Effects of tobacco smoking on cardiovascular disease. Circulation Journal. 2019; 83(10): 1980-5.

25) Kojima G, Iliffe S, Walters K. Smoking as a predictor of frailty: a systematic review. BMC Geriatr. 2015; 15: 131.

26) Messner B, Bernhard D. Smoking and Cardiovascular Disease. Arteriosclerosis, Thrombosis, and Vascular Biology. 2014; 34 (3): 509-15.

27) Mukamal KJ, Rimm EB. Alcohol's effects on the risk for coronary heart disease. Alcohol Res Health. 2001; 25 (4): 255-61.

28) Piano MR. Alcohol's Effects on the Cardiovascular System. Alcohol Res. 2017; 38 (2): 219-41.

29) Soltani S, Jayedi A, Ghoreishy S, Mousavirad M, Movahed S, Jabbari M, et al. Alcohol consumption and frailty risk: a dose–response meta-analysis of cohort studies. Age and Ageing. 2024; 53 (9).

30) Ortolá R, García-Esquinas E, León-Muñoz LM, Guallar-Castillón P, Valencia-Martín JL, Galán I, et al. Patterns of Alcohol Consumption and Risk of Frailty in Community-dwelling Older Adults. J Gerontol A Biol Sci Med Sci. 2016; 71 (2): 251-8.

31) Kojima G, Jivraj S, Iliffe S, Falcaro M, Liljas A, Walters K. Alcohol Consumption and Risk of Incident Frailty: English Longitudinal Study of Aging. J Am Med Dir Assoc. 2019; 20 (6): 725-9.

32) Australian Institute of Health Welfare. Chronic conditions and multimorbidity. Canberra: AIHW; 2022.

33) National Center for Chronic Disease Prevention and Health Promotion 2023; Pages: https:// www.cdc.gov/ chronicdisease/resources/ infographic/ chronic-diseases.htm.

34) Bhattarai U, Bashyal B, Shrestha A, Koirala B, Sharma SK. Frailty and chronic diseases: A bi-directional relationship. Aging Medicine. 2024; 7 (4): 510-5.

35) Sinclair AJ, Rodriguez-Mañas L. Diabetes and Frailty: Two Converging Conditions? Canadian Journal of Diabetes. 2016; 40 (1): 77-83.

36) Wu Y, Xiong T, Tan X, Chen L. Frailty and risk of microvascular complications in patients with type 2 diabetes: a population-based cohort study. BMC Medicine. 2022; 20 (1): 473.

37) Morley JE, Malmstrom TK, Rodriguez-Mañas L, Sinclair AJ. Frailty, sarcopenia and diabetes. J Am Med Dir Assoc. 2014; 15 (12): 853-9.

38) Vetrano DL, Palmer KM, Galluzzo L, Giampaoli S, Marengoni A, Bernabei R, et al. Hypertension and frailty: a systematic review and meta-analysis. BMJ Open. 2018; 8 (12): e024406.

39) Luo D, Cheng Y, Zhang H, Ba M, Chen P, Li H, et al. Association between high blood pressure and long-term cardiovascular events in young adults: systematic review and meta-analysis. BMJ. 2020; 370: m3222.

40) Aprahamian I, Sassaki E, Dos Santos MF, Izbicki R, Pulgrossi RC, Biella MM, et al. Hypertension and frailty in older adults. J Clin Hypertens (Greenwich). 2018; 20(1): 186-92.

41) Cosimo Marcello B, Maria Domenica A, Gabriele P, Elisa M, Francesca B. Lifestyle and Hypertension: An Evidence-Based Review. Journal of Hypertension and Management. 2018; 4 (1).

42) Lavie CJ, Milani RV, Ventura HO. Obesity and cardiovascular disease: risk factor, paradox, and impact of weight loss. J Am Coll Cardiol. 2009; 53 (21): 1925-32.

43) Yuan L, Chang M, Wang J. Abdominal obesity, body mass index and the risk of frailty in community-dwelling

older adults: a systematic review and meta-analysis. Age and Ageing. 2021; 50 (4): 1118-28.

44) Powell-Wiley TM, Poirier P, Burke LE, Després J-P, Gordon-Larsen P, Lavie CJ, et al. Obesity and Cardiovascular Disease: A Scientific Statement From the American Heart Association. Circulation. 2021;143 (21): e984-e1010.

45) Polyzos SA, Margioris AN. Sarcopenic obesity. Hormones (Athens). 2018; 17 (3): 321-31.

46) Correa R, Wayar F, Reaven P, Corpas E. Chapter 19 - Dyslipidemia in the Elderly. In: Corpas E, ed. Endocrinology of Aging: Elsevier; 2021: 607-50.

47) Hu Y, Wang X, Lin L, Huan J, Li Y, Zhang L, et al. Association of remnant cholesterol with frailty: findings from observational and Mendelian randomization analyses. Lipids in Health and Disease. 2023; 22 (1): 115.

48) Yin M, Zhang X, Zheng X, Chen C, Tang H, Yu Z, et al. Cholesterol alone or in combination is associated with frailty among community-dwelling older adults: A cross-sectional study. Exp Gerontol. 2023; 180: 112254.

49) Motta F, Sica A, Selmi C. Frailty in Rheumatic Diseases. Frontiers in Immunology. 2020; 11.

50) Cook MJ, Verstappen SMM, Lunt M, O'Neill TW. Increased Frailty in Individuals With Osteoarthritis and Rheumatoid Arthritis and the Influence of Comorbidity: An Analysis of the UK Biobank Cohort. Arthritis Care & Research. 2022; 74 (12): 1989-96.

51) Arthritis Foundation; Pages: https://www.arthritis.org/health-wellness/about-arthritis /related-conditions/ other-diseases/arthritis-and-heart-disease on 23 December 2024.

52) Hannan M, Chen J, Hsu J, Zhang X, Saunders MR, Brown J, et al. Frailty and Cardiovascular Outcomes in Adults With CKD: Findings From the Chronic Renal Insufficiency Cohort (CRIC) Study. Am J Kidney Dis. 2024; 83 (2): 208-15.

53) Kennard A, Glasgow N, Rainsford S, Talaulikar G. Frailty in chronic kidney disease: challenges in nephrology practice. A review of current literature. Internal Medicine Journal. 2023; 53 (4): 465-72.

54) Wang L, Zhang X, Liu X. Prevalence and clinical impact of frailty in COPD: a systematic review and meta-analysis. BMC Pulmonary Medicine. 2023; 23 (1): 164.

55) Peter H, James L, Jennifer KQ, Bhautesh DJ, Barbara IN, David AM, et al. Frailty in COPD: an analysis of prevalence and clinical impact using UK Biobank. BMJ Open Respiratory Research. 2022; 9 (1): e001314.

56) Wang Z, Hu X, Dai Q. Is it possible to reverse frailty in patients with chronic obstructive pulmonary disease? Clinics. 2020; 75: e1778.

57) Lahousse L, Ziere G, Verlinden VJ, Zillikens MC, Uitterlinden AG, Rivadeneira F, et al. Risk of Frailty in Elderly With COPD: A Population-Based Study. J Gerontol A Biol Sci Med Sci. 2016; 71 (5): 689-95.

58) Ekram ARMS, Tonkin AM, Ryan J, Beilin L, Ernst ME, Espinoza SE, et al. The association between frailty and incident cardiovascular disease events in community-dwelling healthy older adults. Am Heart J Plus. 2023; 28.

59) Panayi AC, Orkaby AR, Sakthivel D, Endo Y, Varon D, Roh D, et al. Impact of frailty on outcomes in surgical patients: A systematic review and meta-analysis. Am J Surg. 2019; 218 (2): 393-400.

60) Ekram ARMS, Woods RL, Britt C, Espinoza S, Ernst ME, Ryan J. The Association Between Frailty and All-Cause Mortality in Community-Dwelling Older Individuals: An Umbrella Review. The Journal of Frailty & Aging. 2021; 10 (4): 320-6.

61) Han CY, Miller M, Yaxley A, Baldwin C, Woodman R, Sharma Y. Effectiveness of combined exercise and nutrition interventions in prefrail or frail older hospitalised patients: a systematic review and meta-analysis. BMJ Open. 2020; 10 (12): e040146.

62) Travers J, Romero-Ortuno R, Bailey J, Cooney M-T. Delaying and reversing frailty: a systematic review of primary care interventions. British Journal of General Practice. 2019; 69 (678): e61.

63) Borge CR, Hagen KB, Mengshoel AM, Omenaas E, Moum T, Wahl AK. Effects of controlled breathing exercises and respiratory muscle training in people with chronic obstructive pulmonary disease: results from evaluating the quality of evidence in systematic reviews. BMC Pulmonary Medicine. 2014; 14 (1): 184.

64) Mitnitski A, Rockwood K. Aging as a Process of Deficit Accumulation: Its Utility and Origin. In: Jazwinski SM, Yashin AI, eds. Aging and Health - A Systems Biology Perspective: S. Karger AG; 2014: 0.

65) Mitnitski AB, Mogilner AJ, Rockwood K. Accumulation of deficits as a proxy measure of aging. Scientific World Journal. 2001; 1: 323-36.

66) Dent E, Kowal P, Hoogendijk EO. Frailty measurement in research and clinical practice: A review. European Journal of Internal Medicine. 2016; 31: 3-10.

67) Wannamethee SG. Frailty and increased risk of cardiovascular disease: are we at a crossroad to include frailty in cardiovascular risk assessment in older adults? European Heart Journal. 2021; 43 (8): 827-9.

68) Australian Institute of Health and Welfare. Heart, stroke and vascular disease: Australian facts. Canberra: AIHW; 2024.

69) Knuuti J, Wijns W, Saraste A, Capodanno D, Barbato E, Funck-Brentano C, et al. 2019 ESC Guidelines for the diagnosis and management of chronic coronary syndromes. Eur Heart J. 2020; 41 (3): 407-77.

70) Torpy JM, Burke AE, Glass RM. JAMA patient page. Coronary heart disease risk factors. Jama. 2009; 302 (21): 2388.

71) Veronese N, Cereda E, Stubbs B, Solmi M, Luchini C, Manzato E, et al. Risk of cardiovascular disease morbidity and mortality in frail and pre-frail older adults: Results from a meta-analysis and exploratory meta-regression analysis. Ageing Res Rev. 2017; 35: 63-73.

72) Damluji AA, Chung S-E, Xue Q-L, Hasan RK, Forman DE, Batchelor W, et al. Abstract 16418: Physical Frailty Phenotype and Development of Geriatric Syndromes in Older Adults With Coronary Heart Disease. Circulation. 2020; 142 (Suppl_3): A16418-A.

73) Tchalla A, Laubarie-Mouret C, Cardinaud N, Gayot C, Rebiere M, Dumoitier N, et al. Risk factors of frailty and functional disability in community-dwelling older adults: a cross-sectional analysis of the FREEDOM-LNA cohort study. BMC Geriatrics. 2022; 22 (1): 762.

74) Talha KM, Pandey A, Fudim M, Butler J, Anker SD, Khan MS. Frailty and heart failure: State-of-the-art review. Journal of Cachexia, Sarcopenia and Muscle. 2023; 14 (5): 1959-72.

75) Zhang Y, Yuan M, Gong M, Tse G, Li G, Liu T. Frailty and Clinical Outcomes in Heart Failure: A Systematic Review and Meta-analysis. J Am Med Dir Assoc. 2018; 19 (11): 1003-8.e1.

76) MacEachern E, Quach J, Giacomantonio N, Theou O, Hillier T, Abel-Adegbite I, et al. Cardiac rehabilitation and frailty: a systematic review and meta-analysis. Eur J Prev Cardiol. 2024; 31 (16): 1960-76.

77) Buttery AK. Cardiac Rehab for Frail Older People. Adv Exp Med Biol. 2020; 1216: 131-47.

78) Loewenthal J, Berning MJ, Wayne PM, Eckstrom E, Orkaby AR. Holistic frailty prevention: The promise of movement-based mind-body therapies. Aging Cell. 2024; 23(1): e13986.

79) Damluji AA, Alfaraidhy M, AlHajri N, Rohant NN, Kumar M, Al Malouf C, et al. Sarcopenia and Cardiovascular Diseases. Circulation. 2023; 147 (20): 1534-53.

80) Powell KE, King AC, Buchner DM, Campbell WW, DiPietro L, Erickson KI, et al. The Scientific Foundation for the Physical Activity Guidelines for Americans, 2nd Edition. Journal of Physical Activity and Health;16 (1): 1-11.

81) Abellan van Kan G, Rolland Y, Andrieu S, Bauer J, Beauchet O, Bonnefoy M. Gait speed at usual pace as a predictor of adverse outcomes in community-dwelling older people an International Academy on Nutrition and Aging (IANA) Task Force. J Nutr Health Aging. 2009; 13.

82) Samala RV, Navas V, Saluke E, Ciocon JO. Heart failure in frail, older patients: We can do 'MORE'. Cleveland Clinic Journal of Medicine. 2011; 78 (12): 837.

83) Pavlovic NV, Gilotra NA, Lee CS, Ndumele C, Mammos D, Dennisonhimmelfarb C, et al. Fatigue in Persons With Heart Failure: A Systematic Literature Review and Meta-Synthesis Using the Biopsychosocial Model of Health. Journal of Cardiac Failure. 2022; 28 (2): 283-315.

84) Salmon T, Essa H, Tajik B, Isanejad M, Akpan A, Sankaranarayanan R. The Impact of Frailty and Comorbidities on Heart Failure Outcomes. Cardiac Failure Review 2022; 8: e07. 2022.

85) Yang ZC, Lin H, Jiang GH, Chu YH, Gao JH, Tong ZJ, et al. Frailty Is a Risk Factor for Falls in the Older Adults: A Systematic Review and Meta-Analysis. The journal of nutrition, health & aging. 2023; 27 (6): 487-95.

86) Lettino M, Mascherbauer J, Nordaby M, Ziegler A, Collet JP, Derumeaux G, et al. Cardiovascular disease in the elderly: proceedings of the European Society of Cardiology—Cardiovascular Round Table. European Journal of Preventive Cardiology. 2022; 29 (10): 1412-24.

87) Anker SD, Coats AJS. Exercise for Frail, Elderly Patients with Acute Heart Failure — A Strong Step Forward. New England Journal of Medicine. 2021; 385 (3): 276-7.

88) Vitale C, Uchmanowicz I. Frailty in patients with heart failure. European Heart Journal Supplements. 2019; 21 (Supplement_L): L12-L6.

89) Winzer EB, Woitek F, Linke A. Physical Activity in the Prevention and Treatment of Coronary Artery Disease. Journal of the American Heart Association;7 (4): e007725.

90) Tapsell LC, Neale EP, Probst Y. Dietary Patterns and Cardiovascular Disease: Insights and Challenges for Considering Food Groups and Nutrient Sources. Curr Atheroscler Rep. 2019; 21(3): 9.

91) Aune D, Giovannucci E, Boffetta P, Fadnes LT, et al. Fruit and vegetable intake and the risk of cardiovascular disease, total cancer and all-cause mortality-a systematic review and dose-response meta-analysis of prospective studies. Int J Epidemiol. 2017; 46 (3): 1029-56.

92) Khan SU, Lone AN, Khan MS, Virani SS, et al. Effect of omega-3 fatty acids on cardiovascular outcomes: A systematic review and meta-analysis. eClinicalMedicine. 2021; 38.

93) Lorenzo-López L, Maseda A, de Labra C, Regueiro-Folgueira L, Rodríguez-Villamil JL, Millán-Calenti JC. Nutritional determinants of frailty in older adults: A systematic review. BMC Geriatrics. 2017; 17 (1): 108.

94) Nwadiugwu MC. Frailty and the Risk of Polypharmacy in the Older Person: Enabling and Preventative Approaches. J Aging Res. 2020; 2020: 6759521.

95) Sinnott C, Bradley CP. Multimorbidity or polypharmacy: two sides of the same coin? J Comorb. 2015; 5: 29-31.

96) Masnoon N, Shakib S, Kalisch-Ellett L, Caughey GE. What is polypharmacy? A systematic review of definitions. BMC geriatrics. 2017; 17 (1): 230.

97) Mehta RS, Kochar BD, Kennelty K, Ernst ME, Chan AT. Emerging approaches to polypharmacy among older adults. Nature Aging. 2021; 1 (4): 347-56.

98) Liacos M, Page AT, Etherton-Beer C. Deprescribing in older people. Australian Prescriber. 2020; 43 (4) : 114-20.

99) Hiriscau EI, Bodolea C. The Role of Depression and Anxiety in Frail Patients with Heart Failure. Diseases. 2019; 7 (2).

100) Vaughan L, Corbin AL, Goveas JS. Depression and frailty in later life: a systematic review. Clin Interv Aging. 2015; 10: 1947-58.

101) Buigues C, Padilla-Sánchez C, Garrido JF, Navarro-Martínez R, Ruiz-Ros V, Cauli O. The relationship between depression and frailty syndrome: a systematic review. Aging Ment Health. 2015; 19 (9): 762-72.

102) Hawkley LC, Thisted RA, Cacioppo JT. Loneliness predicts reduced physical activity: cross-sectional & longitudinal analyses. Health Psychol. 2009; 28 (3): 354-63.

103) Takatori K, Matsumoto D. Social factors associated with reversing frailty progression in community-dwelling late-stage elderly people: An observational study. PLoS One. 2021; 16 (3): e0247296.

104) McHugh JE, Dowling M, Butler A, Lawlor BA. Psychological distress and frailty transitions over time in community-dwelling older adults. Ir J Psychol Med. 2016; 33 (2): 111-9.

105) Wallcraft J. Holistic approaches in mental health. Learning about Mental Health Practice. 2008: 555-70.

106) Arakelyan S, Mikula-Noble N, Ho L, Lone N, Anand A, Lyall MJ, et al. Effectiveness of holistic assessment-based interventions for adults with multiple long-term conditions and frailty: an umbrella review of systematic reviews. The Lancet Healthy Longevity. 2023; 4 (11): e629-e44.

107) Mishra SK, Togneri E, Tripathi B, Trikamji B. Spirituality and Religiosity and Its Role in Health and Diseases. Journal of Religion and Health. 2017; 56 (4): 1282-301.

108) Chattu VK, Manzar MD, Kumary S, Burman D, Spence DW, Pandi-Perumal SR. The Global Problem of Insufficient

Sleep and Its Serious Public Health Implications. Healthcare (Basel). 2018; 7 (1).

109) Newman MG, Zainal NH. The value of maintaining social connections for mental health in older people. The Lancet Public Health. 2020; 5 (1): e12-e3.

110) Editorial. Brain and body are more intertwined than we knew. Nature. 2023; 623 (7986): 223-4.

111) Mensah GA, Fuster V. Sex and Gender Differences in Cardiovascular Health. Journal of the American College of Cardiology. 2022; 79 (14): 1385-7.

112) Davis MR, Lee CS, Corcoran A, Gupta N, Uchmanowicz I, Denfeld QE. Gender differences in the prevalence of frailty in heart failure: A systematic review and meta-analysis. International Journal of Cardiology. 2021; 333: 133-40.

113) Tjoe B, Barsky L, Wei J, Samuels B, Azarbal B, Merz CNB, et al. Coronary microvascular dysfunction: Considerations for diagnosis and treatment. Cleveland Clinic Journal of Medicine. 2021; 88 (10): 561.

114) Gaignard SM, Dave EK, Warnock RK, Bortfeld KS, Moncayo VM, Mehta PK. Coronary Microvascular Dysfunction in Women. Current Cardiovascular Risk Reports. 2024;18(6):81-93.

115) Iorga A, Cunningham CM, Moazeni S, Ruffenach G, Umar S, Eghbali M. The protective role of estrogen and estrogen receptors in cardiovascular disease and the controversial use of estrogen therapy. Biology of Sex Differences. 2017; 8 (1): 33.

116) Moolman JA. Unravelling the cardioprotective mechanism of action of estrogens. Cardiovascular Research. 2006; 69 (4): 777-80.

117) Regitz-Zagrosek V. Sex and Gender Differences in Cardiovascular Disease. In: Oertelt-Prigione S, Regitz-Zagrosek V, eds. Sex and Gender Aspects in Clinical Medicine. London: Springer London; 2012: 17-44.

118) EUGenMed T, Group CCS, Regitz-Zagrosek V, Oertelt-Prigione S, Prescott E, Franconi F, et al. Gender in cardiovascular diseases: impact on clinical manifestations, management, and outcomes. European Heart Journal. 2015; 37 (1): 24-34.

119) Nguyen DD, Arnold SV. Impact of frailty on disease-specific health status in cardiovascular disease. Heart. 2023; 109 (13): 977.

120) The L. Cardiology's problem women. The Lancet. 2019; 393 (10175): 959.

121) Maserejian NN, Link CL, Lutfey KL, Marceau LD, McKinlay JB. Disparities in physicians' interpretations of heart disease symptoms by patient gender: results of a video vignette factorial experiment. J Womens Health (Larchmt). 2009; 18 (10): 1661-7.

122) Victor Chang Cardiac Research Institute; Pages: https://www.victorchang.edu.au/heart-disease/ women on 23 December 2024.

123) Rentscher KE, Klopack ET, Crimmins EM, Seeman TE, Cole SW, Carroll JE. Social relationships and epigenetic aging in older adulthood: Results from the Health and Retirement Study. Brain, Behavior, and Immunity. 2023; 114: 349-59.

124) Vila J. Social Support and Longevity: Meta-Analysis-Based Evidence and Psychobiological Mechanisms. Frontiers in Psychology. 2021; 12.

125) Baldasseroni S, Silverii MV, Herbst A, Orso F, Di Bari M, Pratesi A, et al. Predictors of physical frailty improvement in older patients enrolled in a multidisciplinary cardiac rehabilitation program. Heart and Vessels. 2023; 38 (8): 1056-64.

126) Pozzi M, Mariani S, Scanziani M, Passolunghi D, Bruni A, Finazzi A, et al. The frail patient undergoing cardiac surgery: lessons learned and future perspectives. Frontiers in Cardiovascular Medicine. 2023; 10.

127) Wang Y, Wang B. Risk factors of delirium after cardiac surgery: a systematic review and meta-analysis. Journal of Cardiothoracic Surgery. 2024; 19 (1): 675.

128) Liu S, Xiong X-y, Guo T, Xiang Q, Zhang M-j, Sun X-l. Understanding frailty: a qualitative study of older heart failure patients' frail experience and perceptions of healthcare professionals with frailty. BMC Geriatrics. 2024; 24 (1): 1012.

129) Yoong SQ, Tan R, Jiang Y. Dyadic relationships between informal caregivers and older adults with chronic heart failure: a systematic review and meta-synthesis. European Journal of Cardiovascular Nursing. 2024; 23 (8): 833-54.

130) Lie I, Tørris C, Danielsen SO. Informal caregivers and older adults with chronic heart failure: a commentary. European Journal of Cardiovascular Nursing. 2024; 23 (8): e173-e4.

131) Vavasour G, Giggins OM, Doyle J, Kelly D. How wearable sensors have been utilised to evaluate frailty in older adults: a systematic review. Journal of NeuroEngineering and Rehabilitation. 2021; 18 (1): 112.

132) Canali S, Ferretti A, Schiaffonati V, Blasimme A. Wearable Technologies for Healthy Ageing: Prospects, Challenges, and Ethical Considerations. J Frailty & Aging. 2024; 13 (2): 149-56.

133) Fougère B, Vellas B, van Kan GA, Cesari M. Identification of biological markers for better characterization of older subjects with physical frailty and sarcopenia. Transl Neurosci. 2015; 6 (1): 103-10.

134) Ruan Q, D'Onofrio G, Sancarlo D, Greco A, Lozupone M, Seripa D, et al. Emerging biomarkers and screening for cognitive frailty. Aging Clinical and Experimental Research. 2017; 29 (6): 1075-86.

135) El Assar M, Rodriguez-Sanchez I, Álvarez-Bustos A, Rodríguez-Mañas L. Biomarkers of Frailty. In: Ruiz JG, Theou O, eds. Frailty: A Multidisciplinary Approach to Assessment, Management, and Prevention. Cham: Springer International Publishing; 2024: 91-102.

136) Mhlanga D. Artificial Intelligence in Elderly Care: Navigating Ethical and Responsible AI Adoption for Seniors. In: Mhlanga D, Dzingirai M, eds. Fostering Long-Term Sustainable Development in Africa: Overcoming Poverty, Inequality, and Unemployment. Cham: Springer Nature Switzerland; 2024: 411-40.

137) Zhao D, Sun X, Shan B, Yang Z, Yang J, Liu H, et al. Research status of elderly-care robots and safe human-robot interaction methods. Frontiers in Neuroscience. 2023; 17.

138) Cai R, Gao L, Gao C, Yu L, Zheng X, Bennett DA, et al. Circadian disturbances and frailty risk in older adults. Nature Communications. 2023; 14 (1): 7219.

139) Chrysikou E, Biddulph J, Loizides F, Hobbs H. I am frail and my robot is stuck on the corridor: cohabitation of people with frailty and robots. European Journal of Public Health. 2024; 34 (Supplement_3).

140) Morris L, Diteesawat RS, Rahman N, Turton A, Cramp M, Rossiter J. The-state-of-the-art of soft robotics to assist mobility: a review of physiotherapist and patient identified limitations of current lower-limb exoskeletons and the potential soft-robotic solutions. Journal of NeuroEngineering and Rehabilitation. 2023; 20 (1): 18.

141) Cesari M, Bernabei R, Vellas B, Fielding RA, Rooks D, Azzolino D, et al. Challenges in the Development of Drugs for Sarcopenia and Frailty - Report from the International Conference on Frailty and Sarcopenia Research (ICFSR) Task Force. J Frailty Aging. 2022; 11 (2): 135-42.

142) Mahindran E, Law JX, Ng MH, Nordin F. Mesenchymal Stem Cell Transplantation for the Treatment of Age-Related Musculoskeletal Frailty. International Journal of Molecular Sciences. 2021; 22 (19): 10542.

143) Zhu Y, Ge J, Huang C, Liu H, Jiang H. Application of mesenchymal stem cell therapy for aging frailty: from mechanisms to therapeutics. Theranostics. 2021; 11 (12): 5675-85.

BOOKS BY THIS AUTHOR

Frailty Fighters: Steps To A Healthier Aging

Are you ready to age strong, stay sharp, and keep moving with ease for years to come?

"Frailty Fighters: A Guide to a Healthier Aging Journey" is your go-to guide for building resilience from your 20s onward. This book unlocks the science behind why frailty isn't just an "old age" issue —it's a lifelong journey. With practical advice and a light-hearted tone, it shows you how simple habits, set in motion today, can keep you vibrant, flexible, and independent well into your later years.

Discover easy ways to boost muscle strength, protect bone health, and maintain flexibility—no matter your fitness level. Uncover the connections between sleep, nutrition, and heart health and how they each play a role in your aging experience. Explore why social connections, mental resilience, and a balanced lifestyle are just as vital to staving off frailty as physical exercise.

Packed with tips, activities, and fun challenges, "Frailty Fighters: A Guide to a Healthier Aging Journey" is designed to inspire readers from 20 to 50 to make lasting changes for a frailty-free future. Learn how to invest in yourself today so that you can live with confidence and strength tomorrow. Aging is inevitable, but frailty is not. Embrace this empowering journey to health, vitality, and a life well-lived.

Frailty And Nutrition: Powering Resilience

"Frailty and Nutrition: Powering Resilience" is a simple, useful guide that helps you face the challenges of aging with strength and energy. It explains how proper nutrition can boost resilience and fight frailty, focusing on the importance of key nutrients and gut health. With clear advice and practical tips, it shows how to make smart food choices to stay physically, mentally, and socially healthy. Whether you want to prevent frailty or manage it better, this book is a helpful tool for living a healthier, more independent life. Ideal for older adults, caregivers, and anyone who wants to age well.

Frailty And Fitness: The Transformative Power Of Exercise

Frailty often seems like an inevitable companion of aging, but it does not have to be. 'Frailty and Fitness: The Transformative Power of Exercise' is your comprehensive guide to understanding this condition and reclaiming vitality through the power of movement. Packed with practical advice, this book delves into the science of frailty, revealing how targeted exercises can help rebuild strength, improve balance, and restore independence.

From resistance and power training to overcoming barriers and designing personalized programs, this book provides actionable steps for individuals at all levels of fitness. Discover inspiring stories, easy-to-follow exercises, and the latest research on how exercise not only combats physical frailty but also enhances mental and social well-being.

Whether you are an older adult looking to regain confidence or a caregiver aiming to support someone you love, 'Frailty and Fitness: The Transformative Power of Exercise' offers the tools you need to embrace an active, healthy lifestyle. Start small, stay consistent, and watch how even modest efforts can lead to transformative results. Empower yourself to age with strength, resilience, and joy—because it is never too late to rewrite your story.